Be Well

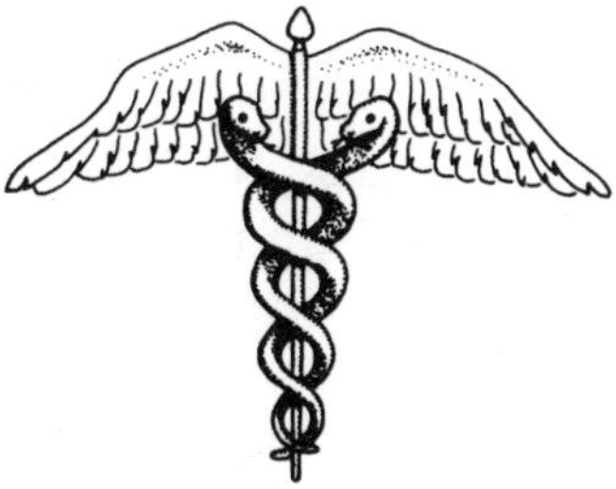

Mike Samuels, M.D.

Hal Z. Bennett

Illustrated by **Susan Ida Smith**

A RANDOM HOUSE • BOOKWORKS BOOK

First printing, September 1974, 7,500 copies in cloth

Illustrations by Susan Ida Smith
Typeset by Vera Allen Composition Service, Hayward, California
(with special thanks to Vera, Jody, Lyn, Betty and Bob)
Printed and bound at Colonial Press, Clinton, Massachusetts
under the direction of Dean Ragland, Random House.

This book is co-published by Random House Inc.
201 East 50th Street
New York, N. Y. 10022

and The Bookworks
2043 Francisco
Berkeley, California 94709

Distributed in the United States by Random House and simultaneously published in Canada by Random House of Canada Limited, Toronto.

Booksellers please order from Random House.

LIBRARY OF CONGRESS CATALOGING IN PUBLICATION DATA:

Samuels, Mike
Be well.

1. Hygiene. 2. Medicine, Popular. I. Bennett, Harold, 1936- II. Title.
RA776.S2813 613 74-8134
ISBN 0-394-49182-3

Manufactured in the United States of America.

''May You Be Well''

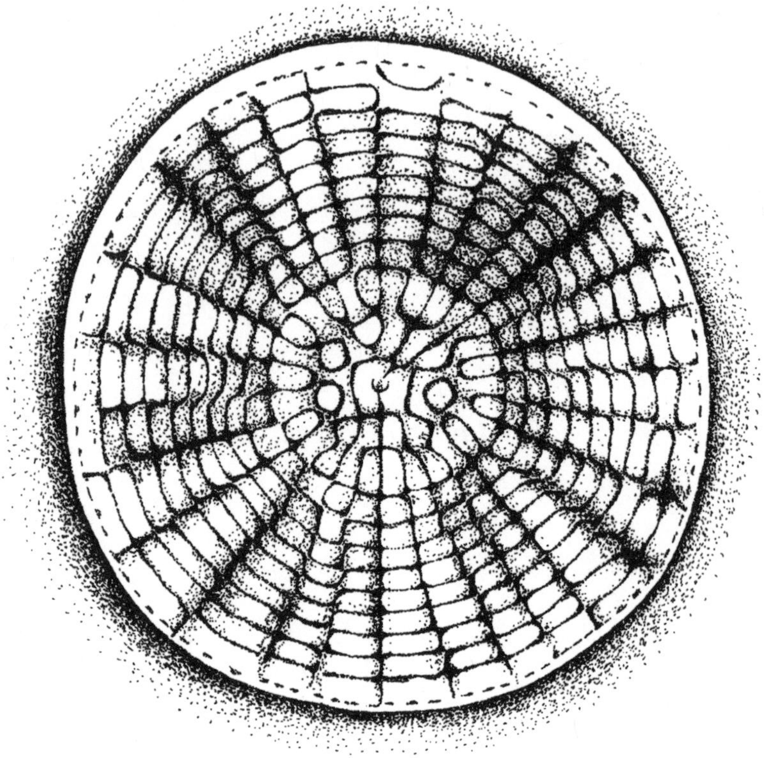

1

You Can Free Yourself To Be Well

Sound waves produced by striking a steel disc

(Turn to page 152 for an explanation of the illustrations.)

At our lectures we always invite people to ask questions. Although each person seems to ask it in a different way, most people want to know, "What can I do about disease in my life?" Our answer begins with this statement:

You can make yourself well by freeing inborn healing abilities which you already possess.

We believe that everyone has these abilities to *be well*. We are each born with these abilities and they are active every moment of our lives. What are these abilities?

Medical scientists have called them "self regulatory processess" or "inborn healing abilities." They include: the human body's antibody system, and the body's other abilities for maintaining optimum heart beat, blood pressure, respiration rate, blood flow, acid-base balance, electro-magnetic properties, and body temperature.

These abilities express themselves in each of us as a natural impulse to be well. It is an impulse to find comfort as opposed to pain, to find ease as opposed to *dis*-ease, to find harmony as opposed to *dis*-harmony.

This impulse toward ease represents a guiding force which is available to us all every moment of our lives and which is manifest in many forms throughout the world in which we live. Physicists, psychologists, students of religion, and doctors have all dealt with the underlying principles of this force. In physics one might see it as a force which keeps electrons spinning in a particular orbit around a nucleus. In psychology one might see it as that part of the human psyche which seeks release from conflict in order to find comfort. In studying religions one might see it as that impulse which has caused human beings, throughout history, to seek peace through union with God. In medicine a doctor might see it as an asthmatic person's desire to find something to help him breathe more comfortably.

You experience this force in your own body when you injure yourself. For example, when you cut your finger, you feel pain. Your impulse is to do something about the cut. Perhaps you stop what you are doing, wash the cut and put on a bandage. Without your having to think about it, your impulse for ease or comfort has guided you to find specific things to do to help your inborn healing abilities work at their best. Your inborn healing abilities, having been freed to work better as a result of your acts, continue to cleanse the wound and create new tissue even as you go on to do other things in your life.

But you may say, "If I have these inborn healing abilities and a natural impulse for ease, why do I get sick?"

The answer is that we all live in ways and do things that obscure our inborn healing abilities and prevent them from working at their best. For example, on our T.V. screens we see a housewife losing her temper with her children, and finding herself with a headache by the time her husband comes home from work. Or we see a businessman pressured as the result of a late delivery, and finding himself with acid indigestion after lunch. These are popularizations of situations similar to experiences which each of us have had. Doctors tell us that headaches, indigestion, ulcers, high blood pressure, and even heart attacks can be caused by *tensions which we create* by the things that we do.

We believe that even when people are doing things that can result in illness, their inborn healing abilities and the desire to find ease continue to be strong forces in their lives. In a way, their thoughts, feelings and actions have temporarily prevented their inborn healing abilities from working at their best. But we continue to find evidence that the impulse for ease and the natural healing abilities are still strong. The housewife with a headache seeks relief from her headache. The businessman seeks relief from his stomach distress.

Just as we can do things to stand in the way of our inborn healing abilities, we can also do things that allow them to work at their best. Examples of these experiences are easy to find. A tired businessman goes to the mountains for a weekend, and comes back feeling relaxed, refreshed and healthy. A retired couple, feeling lonely after a close friend moves away, looks over photographs they have collected of pleasurable moments of their life together and they feel exhilarated and energetic afterwards. A woman telephones a friend who she has not seen for many months and feels relaxed and at peace with herself for the rest of the day. Each of these people, wanting to find ease, literally creates, through his or her actions, a relaxed and healthy state in which the body's inborn healing abilities and self-regulatory processes work at their best.

But Scientists have demonstrated that you do not have to be dependent on outside events, such as going on a vacation, or looking at photos, or calling a friend, to relax you or put you at ease. You can deliberately create these relaxed and healthy states *using your mind*. Many of the ways they have demonstrated to be useful are simple extensions of things that you do every day of your life.

"What are these things and how can I learn

to use them?'' a person might ask.

That's what BE WELL is all about. It is about recognizing your inborn healing abilities and learning what you can do to free them to work at their best. It is about learning to be well.

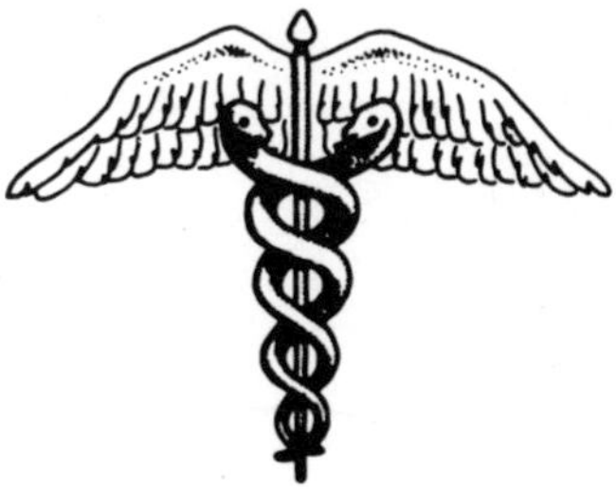

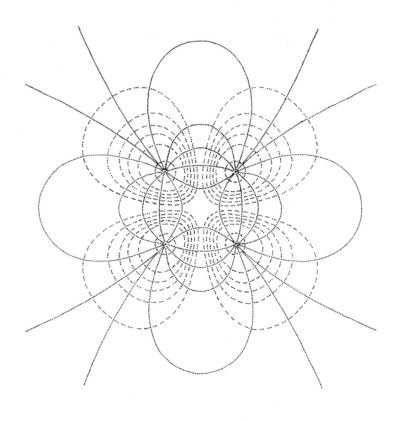

2
Trust Your Feelings

Patterns of force around two positive and two negative charges

Every day you have feelings about the events taking place in your life. These feelings can tell you when your inborn healing abilities and self-regulatory processes are working at their best. When they are working at their best, you feel good. Your body feels comfortable. Your mind feels at peace. Similarly, your feelings can tell you when your abilities are not working at their best. At such times, you feel distressed. Your body feels uncomfortable. Your mind feels distracted.

If you imagine a scale with ease at one end and dis-ease at the other, looking something like this:

EASE					☆			DIS—EASE			
1	2	3	4	5	6	7	8	9	10	11	12

the feelings you experience along the scale range from joy and exhilaration at 1, to pain and suffering at 12. Most of us spend a good part of our lives in the center of the scale, with occasional movements back and forth between right and left ends. Around 5 to 7 we find feelings which are commonplace. These may be anything from a feeling that "things are okay" to a feeling that "things are not quite right." Around 8 are mild dis-eases, such as minor skin rashes, a sore muscle, or a runny nose.

Your feelings of ease and dis-ease can tell you whether or not a particular idea you have or action you take will result in greater ease or dis-ease in your life. These feelings may seem to come from a part of your body, or from your mind. They can be anything from the sensation of "butterflies" in your stomach while you are waiting for an interview to a pleasant and exciting idea about going to the seashore for a vacation, where you have enjoyed yourself in the past.

A feeling of ease of dis-ease can be tension in your shoulders while waiting in bumper-to-bumper commuter traffic; or warmth and relaxation in your muscles following a game of tennis; or general feelings of joy upon meeting someone you love; or an idea that a particular food would be good for dinner; or an idea that you would like to move to the country.

Feelings of ease and dis-ease probably always involve both body and mind. There is no actual separation between them. A feeling of ease might include a tranquil state of mind along with relaxed muscles throughout your body. However these feelings are manifest, they can be used to help you make choices in your live in the same way that you use knowledge which you learn from a book. For example, a pregnant woman has a craving for more milk in her diet. She feels this craving as mental and physical uneasiness and very mild irritability. She notices that the uneasiness and irritability (feelings of dis-ease) of her cravings disappear and she feels better (feelings of ease) after increasing the amount of milk in her diet. Later, she discusses this with her physician, who agrees that the woman's choice was a good one. The physician tells the woman that scientific research has shown how pregnant women often need an increased amount of calcium, and that this additional calcium can come from drinking more milk.

Using your feelings of ease and dis-ease to help you make choices may at first seem quite different than what you have done in the past. Most of us have been taught to trust information collected by other people: by doctors, scientists, teachers, parents, or friends. It is often a great temptation to trust other people's descriptions of their experiences or their data, which they have collected, more than you trust your own feelings.

The process of learning to trust your feelings is accumulative. At first the feelings you notice may be as subtle as mild tension in your shoulders or a feeling that you would like to rest after work. And you may doubt that these feelings are in any way significant. But you act on your feelings to rest after work and you feel better. You experience how trusting your feelings brought ease into your life. Your confidence in the process increases. Each time you consult your feelings in making new choices, you find yourself more receptive to them. As this happens the process becomes clearer and more meaningful to you.

As you read on, you will find yourself accumulating experience and trust in your abilities to make choices using your feelings of ease and disease as your guide. You will begin to experience how choosing actions that bring you ease, or changing situations which cause you to feel disease, will help you be well. You will begin to see how your own feelings are intimately linked with your inborn healing abilities and self-regulating processes.

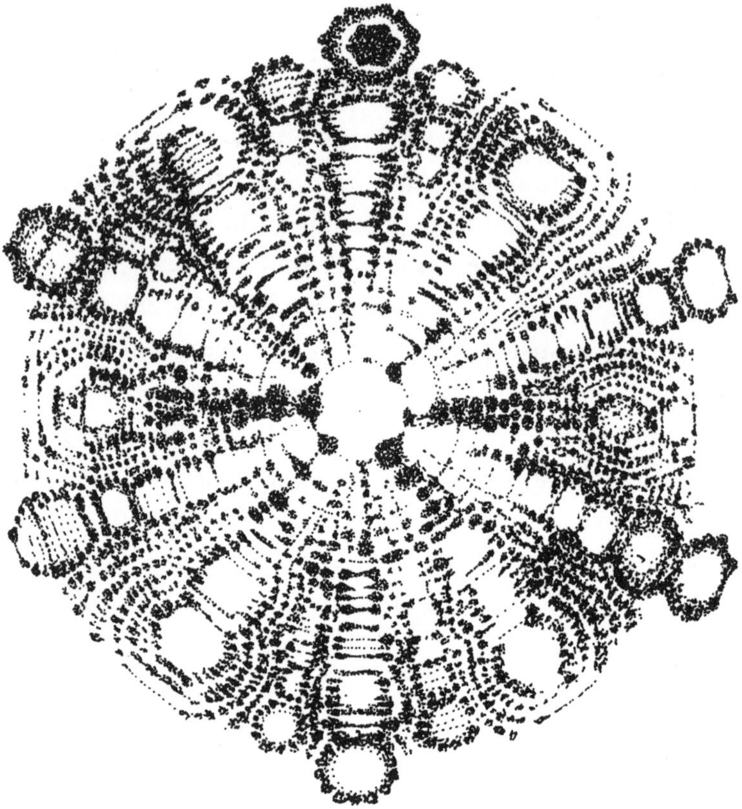

3
Create Your Own World

Tungsten atom magnified about 2 million times

You create your own world. By recognizing how you do this, you gain knowledge to help you make a world in which you can enjoy ease. You need not look far to find evidence for the fact that you do, indeed, create your own world. Let's say that you awaken on the morning of the day you're planning a camping trip to the mountains and, without deliberately doing so, you picture in your mind what kinds of foods you will take along and what you will do to get your equipment ready. Many things may run through your mind as you are doing this. You may remember back to other trips you have taken, recalling how a certain food which you had prepared over a campfire tasted. Or you might remember that you had previously forgotten to take a piece of equipment and you want to make sure to bring it this time. You may also remember how good you felt while you were there. Perhaps you begin to actually experience some of those feelings of pleasure and ease again as you get ready to go.

You plan your route and you picture in your mind the place where you are going. You begin to imagine how you will arrange your camp when you get there. These mental pictures are natural parts of planning the trip. As the day progresses and you act out each part, with perhaps minor variations, you create in the world around you a number of events which, hours before, existed only in your imagination. But this is not a process which is limited to special plans for special occasions.

Without consciously thinking about it we all organize and plan the day ahead as we awaken each morning. As you are getting out of bed and dressing you begin to anticipate experiences you will have that day: meetings which are scheduled; work which excites you and which you want to complete; a drive home with a special friend. In the process of anticipating these things you experience different feelings of ease and dis-ease: tension in your shoulders as you think about an interview you will have; warm, relaxed feelings as you think about a friend you will meet; feelings of peace and self-satisfaction as you think about completing certain jobs. For most people, these early morning feelings come as much milder, *scaled down* versions of feelings which they will have again in the actual experience later in the day.

These processes take place in the simplest events. For example, as lunch time approaches, you begin to feel hungry. Your hunger pangs seem to arouse thoughts, feelings and mental pictures of food. You might imagine yourself going to the kitchen or to a restaurant to prepare or buy food. You might imagine how a certain food looks and tastes. You may even picture yourself sitting down to eat.

By the time you start eating, you have probably forgotten that you first created this experience in your mind. Most people go through these processes automatically while they are working or talking with other people. Few of us are aware that we usually plan our activities in this way. But a small amount of introspection will reveal to you that indeed you do create mental pictures of your actions before you give these mental pictures realities in the everyday world.

Your general feelings of well-being likewise help to determine the world you create. For example, you awaken in the morning in high spirits, looking forward to a pleasant day. In this frame of mind you will tend to notice things in the world which support your elevated feelings, and tend not to notice things that do not support your feelings. As you become aware of events which are compatible with your feelings you tend to participate in them rather than choosing to participate in situations which are less compatible. You notice the reflection of the morning light making patterns in the damp street in front of your house. But you tend not to notice the fact that the city has still not repaired the holes in the street. You want to go out to enjoy the morning air; but you are not even tempted to make a telephone call to complain to the city.

As you express your feeling in the presence of other people, they in turn tend to respond in kind. Thus your feelings help create your world in two important ways: You tend to see and select from the world of objects and events around you those which are compatible with the way you feel. You also send your feelings out into the world, through all your expressions, verbal and non-verbal, and you tend to get back responses harmonious with those expressions.

You may argue that there have been times when you've awakened in fine spirits only to be met by a seemingly hostile world over which you felt you had no control. Or, you may have awakened in a foul mood only to happily have your mood changed by some unexpected event. The thing you discover in both of these cases is that you do not create your world in isolation. Everyone creates his or her own world, but there are times when one person's creation seems to dominate another's. For example, a man feels that in his job *someone else* is creating his daily schedules and determining his actions. Another man might have the same job and feel that the schedules and activities he followed during the day felt good; he might even feel that if he were to create his own schedule it would be almost identical to the one he presently follows at work. Furthermore, two people might come together with very different ideas and create a third point of view quite different from the ideas that either of them originally had. Sometimes you will allow another person's creation to influence yours; sometimes others will allow your world to merge with or dominate theirs. Sometimes your two creations merge to become a new creation. In any case, the choice to allow another person's creation to dominate yours can be your own. That choice, too, is part of the world you create for yourself.

Thoughts and feelings of which you may not be fully aware, or which may seem *random*, or *accidental*, also influence the way in which you create your world. For example, a woman with what later became expressed as a natural love for music, could conceivably be born into a family which paid no attention to music. She goes through her whole childhood without developing skills to express her musical feelings.

As this woman grows older she buys records,

goes to concerts, and even chooses musicians for friends. In spite of these clues, which might seem obvious to other people, our hypothetical, musically-underdeveloped person feels at loose ends and unable to choose something satisfying to do with her life. Then one day, by chance, she picks up a musical instrument and tries it out. The experience moves her deeply and she discovers that she can put together a few notes in a pleasing way, almost immediately. She persists in her experimentation and after a number of weeks decides to take lessons. After several lessons she discovers that she possesses what the teacher calls "an ear for music." As she develops her skills in musical expression, through practice, she feels more deeply fulfilled than ever before in her life. She suddenly understands a little more about how her love for music had influenced her in purchasing records, going to concerts, and choosing musicians for friends. As her awareness and abilities expand she gains confidence in herself as a musician and goes on to pursue it as a profession.

It is not so difficult, then, to see how one's world is created from thoughts and feelings. But your body is also a part of your world; there is a way in which you create it, too. This sounds farfetched until you realize that all cells in your body are being constantly replaced by new cells. The lifespans of cells vary anywhere from a few moments to many months. Thus, at the most obvious level, you can influence the *new growth* of cells in your body by the foods you eat, by the soaps and other chemicals you use on your skin and by they kind of physical exercise you get, since all of these have subtle but far-reaching affects on the lives of cells. For example, when Vitamin A is added to the diet of a person who is deficient in it, that person will notice after several days, night vision improving and subtle changes in skin and hair. Or, a person starts using a milder soap than he or she previously used and notices, after a number of weeks, that a skin rash disappears and red, sore skin is replaced by smooth, good-feeling skin. Or, a person increases his or her daily exercise and, after a week or two, feels stronger and healthier; this good feeling comes as a result of developing new muscle tissue.

Just as Vitamin A, soap or exercise affect

your body, so your thoughts and feelings affect it too. For example, sexual feelings about a person you love, though they take place in your mind when that person is absent from your life, produce physiological changes in your body. For a woman, blood flow is redirected in the mucous membranes of her vagina, resulting in increased moisture there. Similar blood flow changes cause the man's penis to erect.

Blushing is another example of mind affecting body. For example, a feeling or a thought which you have is excited by something your friend says or does. In response, your mind sends messages out through nerve cells in your brain and down through capillaries carrying blood to your skin. These capillaries open and blood rushes to your cheeks, causing the characteristic redness of blushing.

If you relax for a moment by enjoying a deep yawn or sigh, you can immediately experience subtle changes taking place in your body. Sighing and yawning are activities we have all done throughout our lives without thinking too much about them. But they are also natural tools which change your body physiology. The yawn brings extra oxygen into you lungs, momentarily takes brain wave activity to a restful and receptive state, and changes blood flow. When you are tired the reflex to yawn is your body's way of revitalizing tired cells.

If you follow your yawn or sigh by imagining yourself resting quietly and peacefully on a bed, your brain sends signals throughout your body to relax. You begin to feel your muscles actually relax. Just as your mind can cause your muscles to tense, so it can also cause them to relax. Most of us take for granted our ability to tense our muscles, and understand what this ability can accomplish: lifting, walking, and performing hundreds of physical acts each day. But the ability to relax our muscles, though we don't particularly think about it, accomplishes changes at least as important as tension does. Through relaxation, small blood vessels open and carry increased nutrients, hormones, and antibodies to your cells to revitalize them. Relaxing frees your inborn healing abilities to work at their best. In these simple everyday acts you can voluntarily initiate changes in your body through your mind.

By reading the paragraph below you can experience another way in which your mind can affect your physiology:

Simply imagine that you are walking down a busy street in a large city. It is a bright, clear summer day. You go into a large building and enter the elevator. Alone in the elevator, you push the button for the 20th floor. The doors shut. You feel sudden pressure under your feet as the elevator starts to climb. Your stomach flutters as a dial over the door climbs through the numbers from 1 to 20. At last the arrow stops at 20 and the doors open. You take a few steps out and realize that you're on the roof of the building. Curious, you walk over to a low wall and lean over. Far down in the street people appear to be no larger than ants. And the cars moving through the streets look like toys.

When you read the description of the elevator ride, you may feel giddy and flushed, and you may notice slight changes in your breathing and the rate of your heart beat. For some people these bodily changes will be recognized as "feelings of fear" that seem to be located in their stomach; most people refer to them as "butterflies.'' When you imagined yourself on the roof looking down you probably had increased muscular tension in your legs, arms, back and chest. You may have also noticed different sensations in your wrists, hands, feet, or in other parts of your body.

When you imagine yourself on the elevator ride, then up on the roof looking down, you mentally recreate an experience which in real life causes people to be afraid. The changes which take place in your body, as feelings of fear, constitute what biologists call ''the fight and flight syndrome.'' Although you haven't actually been in the dangerous situation which would warrant your body's reactions, the mental image you created discharged nerve cells in your brain in the same way they would be discharged if you had faced real danger. Then, fibers connected to your cerebrum carry signals to your *hypothalmus*. From your hypothalmus, deep within your brain, fibers carry signals to your adrenal glands, over your kidneys. These glands release *epinephrine*, a hormone which opens certain blood vessels and closes others. As a result blood flow is redirected in your body, with some areas getting less than previously while others more.

☆ ☆ ☆

We have discussed in this chapter how thoughts and feelings which take place in your mind can result in actual changes taking place in your body physiology and in events in the wrold around you. Thoughts and feelings about a trip to the mountains result in an actual trip taking place. Feelings of joy and exhilaration upon awakening in the morning result in a person participating in events which they found harmonious with their feelings. Yawning, then imagining yourself resting, resulted in your muscles actually relaxing and your body's cells becoming revitalized. Imagining an elevator ride resulted in hormonal changes in your body.

Sometimes, in your life, you may feel that you deliberately choose the thoughts and feelings which you have, and sometimes you seem hardly aware of any choice being available. But in either case your thoughts and feelings do influence your life. By learning to recognize the power of your thoughts and feelings you place yourself in the position of being able to choose the kind of life you want. You can choose to concentrate on thoughts and feelings that result in dis-ease. Or you can choose to concentrate on thoughts and feelings that result in ease-thoughts and feelings that free your inborn healing abilities to work at their best.

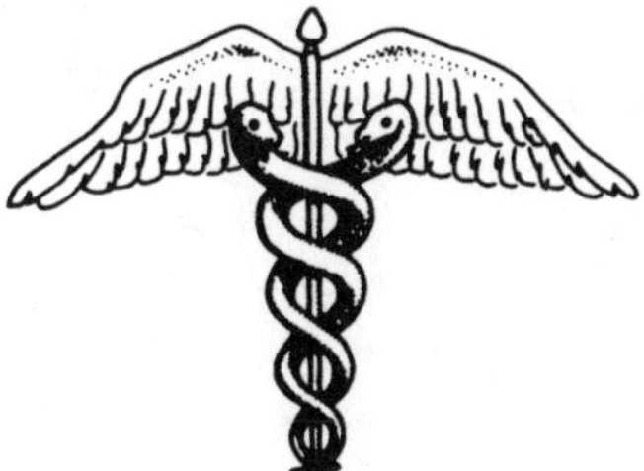

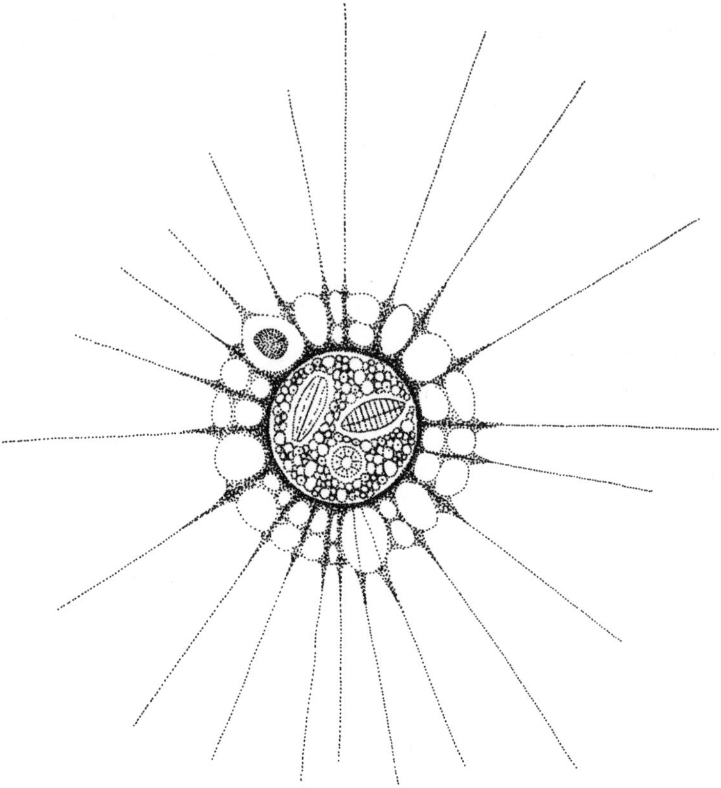

4
Your Universal Self

A one-celled animal, called Actinosphaerium, magnified about 500 times

Imagine going out on a dark night, perhaps with a telescope, and looking up at the stars. Far out past our own planet you see specks of light which scientists tell us have substance just as our own planet has substance. You look further, trying to imagine a beginning or an end to space. As far as you can tell (indeed, as far as the *scientists* have been able to determine) there is none. There seems to be an end to the planets and stars but no end to space itself. You seek for some way to describe, to put into words all and everything which you see, imagine or in some other way recognize as part of our experience. You want some word that will stand not only for what you *can* see but also for things which you can't see: forces of order which cause planets to move around the sun; forces of order which cause things to be born and die; forces which account for the order of the seasons, tides, and the revolution of planets on their poles; and the *life* force itself. Some people have words for these phenomena, others have feelings. In this book, our words to describe "all and everything" are *universe* or *universal order*.

These universal forces are at work in the human body, and are what medical scientists study. The same force that sends molecules spinning around a nucleus and planets around the sun is also manifest in your own body as a particular heart beat, respiration rate, acid-base balance, electromagnetic field for each cell, reproduction rate, growth rate — all these and more. We call this part of you, which regulates your physiology, the "universal self." This self is a kind of personification of your body's inborn healing abilities and self-regulatory principles.

When it is personified in this way, it emphasizes the fact that it is *a part of you* over which you *can* have control.

Your feelings of ease and dis-ease can tell you when you are allowing your universal self the freedom to maintain your body in a well state. You need not look far to find evidence for this: you answer the phone one day and a friend asks you to meet him or her for lunch. You pause, hardly recognizing that you are doing so since it is for no more than a fraction of a second. During that pause, you feel a rush of excited, happy feelings; you feel good, relaxed and comfortable. You accept the invitation. On the way to meet your friend you recall past meetings; you remember that you enjoyed discussing your plans for moving to your new home, and that you both had enjoyed a favorite food. For the rest of that day, you had felt relaxed, warm and high.

In the fractional part of a second after you first heard you friend's voice on the phone, that very brief rush of good feelings told you that you were allowing your universal self the freedom to maintain your body in a well state. The feelings were messages from your universal self. Your acceptance of your friend's invitation was a direct response to that message.

Your universal self is always within you, yet you are more aware of it at some times than at others. The world you create through your actions can obscure this universal self, just as you can obscure some memories of childhood by the busy concerns of adulthood. Or, you can create a world in which your universal self is given freedom, by listening to it each day. As you do this, the expressions of your universal self become increasingly clear and strong.

If you have ever walked through the fog early in the morning, over a path that you know well, you have in your mind an image that illustrates the idea of an obscured but emerging universal self. In the early morning the fog is like a beautiful, silvery screen as the shadows of familiar objects move behind it. The interplay of shapes and shadows entertains you as you move. Then through the silvery screen you see a gray shadow against the horizon which you recognize as the silhouette of a tree. You move toward it and as you do you see the branches of the tree more clearly. Soon you are standing close enough to touch a branch. Even in the dim light you can see the beginnings of buds on the small twigs.

Walking across the foggy meadow and seeing the tree become clearer is similar to discovering your universal self. The tree, or universal self, is always there but it becomes more and more clear to you only as, by your own efforts, you move closer to it.

Let's look at another example of observing the universal self: you might get a call from another person inviting you to lunch, and in the fractional part of a second before you accept or reject their invitation you find that you feel tense, annoyed and ambivalent. However, the feelings in this fractional second do not seem so important to you because this person has been a friend for many years and has done you many favors. You accept the invitation. Then, while on your way to meet him or her you recall the past several times you had lunch together. In each case this person had been late, leaving you to wait alone in the restaurant. You remember the service in the restaurant had seemed poor and you had left feeling aggravated and troubled. Later you may have even suffered from mild indigestion. In this example you did not listen to the messages which came to you as feelings of tension, annoyance and ambivalence, in the fractional part of a second after first receiving the luncheon invitation. Instead, you acted from a part of yourself which reminded you that the person who invited you had been a friend for many years and had done you many favors.

In the examples of both luncheon invitations, the feelings you experienced in the brief pause after hearing your friend's voice were guides which you could use to help you choose actions toward creating your world. They were messages directing you toward creating a world of harmony and ease which would result in a state of well-being. Although these messages took place in only a fraction of a second they were condensations of millions of pieces of information, registering which parts of your body were in harmony, and which parts were not.

By creating an imagined experience (like the elvator ride), you can explore some of the messages which come through in pauses like the ones we've just discussed. As you read through the following paragraph you will automatically create, in your mind, an experience to fully explore in this way:

After a deep yawn, imagine yourself resting on a bed. Then take yourself back to the memory of a particularly happy moment of your life. Remember moments during vacations you have enjoyed, accomplishments in a hobby or exciting challenges in your work, events such as marriage, birth or moving into a new home. Remember experiences of solitude: prayer, meditation, or when you got an insight which changed your life. Remember where the experience took place, whether it was indoors or out. Often it helps to remember an object or a particular sight which was part of the original experience — furnishings of a room or natural surroundings outside. Or you might remember how it felt to spend time there with a friend.

As you let yourself go back into your memories in this way, your experience becomes one of pleasure. Your feelings are in the range of ease. More specifically, one or many parts of your body will feel pleasant; often sensations of warmth, "open-ness," and pleasant tingling can be experienced. These may occur in your ankles, legs, pelvis, abdomen, chest, neck, arms, face, scalp, or any other part of your body. You may notice that your muscles relax, your breathing slows and your heartbeat becomes very calm.

During the same time that this pleasant memory allows you to enjoy messages from your body, you are also receiving messages in the form of ideas and feelings. These messages may seem to come as generalized feelings of well-being such as exhilaration, joy, excitement, love or peace. Even though *generalized*, they may seem to come from one or more organs in the body, such as your eyes, mouth, heart, abdomen, pelvis, legs or arms. From such experiences come the use of expressions like *light-hearted, sexy, delicious, or a-sight-for-sore eyes,* to describe overall feelings we enjoy in situations which please us.

The following narrative is one person's way of describing their feelings after remembering a moment of pleasure:

"I am remembering being in the mountains last year. I had been climbing all day and then came to a wide shelf, where I rested. There was a beautiful view of the valley I'd come from, and the sky was deep blue with a few streaks of clouds.

I pulled off my shirt and shoes and lay there in the sun with a slight breeze blowing over me. I feel that way now . . .

"My muscles feel relaxed, especially in my chest, which also feels warm and tingly. In fact, I feel a general mild tingling all over. My breathing is slow, easy, and rhythmic. My heart beat is slow but it is also even and strong. My whole body feels light and I am hardly aware of it except that it is taking care of itself nicely. I feel exhilarated and joyful, very much at peace with myself. The feelings seem to be coming from my heart and head, and those parts of me feel warm and light."

You begin to realize that the experience of *feeling good* is an expression of many events taking place in your body. It is ease. It is harmony. It is your muscles relaxing, allowing blood to flow freely to all areas, encouraging nutrients, antibodies, hormones, and white blood cells to travel to every part of your body where they are needed. The optimum temperature, acid-base balance and electrical fields can manifest themselves in this state. When you create the experience of feeling good, you turn your body over to the self-regulatory processes, to the universal self, which produces harmony and an optimum state of health. This is the state of *being well*, a state in which your inborn healing abilities can be most strongly effective.

Sometimes it is difficult to experience or to remember feeling good. At such times feelings of discomfort can also be used as guides to help you create the world you want. We have learned to look upon any discomfort as a signal telling us to *seek outside the options which we presently see.* Often this proves to mean that we should lay low and let things pass for the time being. After doing so we later find more opportunity to use our energy to create a world in which *feeling good* can be a reality.

Because experiences of discomfort in which you feel dis-ease are valuable guides in your life it is important to look upon them with a calm mind just as you would an experience of feeling good. The following description of one person's feelings of discomfort, while remembering a difficult situation, helps to demonstrate why this is so:

". . . I was getting into my car to go to work and I suddenly realized that I felt sort of uneasy and up-tight. Things were going pretty well for me in general so I asked myself what started me feeling this way. I remembered, then, that I'd been interrupted at dinner by a phone call the night before. It was Donald telling me that an important order I had taken was going to be a month late. I knew this would hold up my customer's contract schedules. So I was going to have to call my customer and tell him about it, and I knew he wasn't going to like it."

When this person described his feelings, he did so in this way:

"My whole body feels tense. I am hunching my back slightly. My neck aches, and my chin is thrust forward, My thighs and stomach muscles are a little cramped. My chest feels tight, too, and I am breathing in a sort of strained way that isn't the way I usually breathe. I guess my heart is beating a little harder than usual. In my head I'm feeling slightly confused, not knowing exactly what I want to do next."

A feeling of discomfort is a condensation of many events taking place in the body. Muscular tension clamps down blood vessels, slowing the flow of blood and thereby preventing cells from getting their necessary supplies of nutrients, antibodies and hormones; also, waste products build up around cells because normal blood flow, necessary for the normal bathing and cleansing of each cell, is slowed. This produces changes in body temperature, acid-base balance, and electrical fields around cells . . . all contributing to the creation of a good environment for bacteria and virus to multiply. Discomfort is a state in which the universal self and the self-regulatory principles are unable to function at their best. This disharmonious state, maintained over a long period of time, is the state in which illness is most likely to occur.

To develop the experience of feeling good as a tool for making choices and decisions to *be well*, you can develop what we call the "feeling pause." This is the moment between the time a possibility is presented to you and the time you act upon it. One person described it as "that moment when I stop whatever I'm doing, scratch my head, and wonder about what I'm going to do next." In the previously discussed examples of the luncheon invitations, it was the moment between the time that you received the invitation and the moment you accepted or rejected it.

What happens during the feeling pause is this: you relax yourself long enough to explore how your body feels. These feelings, which you detect as ease or dis-ease, comfort or discomfort, relaxation or tension, indicate to you how to make a choice that will be in harmony with your universal self.

To get in touch with your feelings of ease of dis-ease you need only pause and ask yourself how each part of your body feels from time to time throughout the day. For example, after finishing a telephone call, you pause. You may close your eyes for better concentration. Then you ask yourself how you feel: good, bad, comfortable, uncomfortable, happy, unhappy, at ease or ill-at-ease? Then feel the sensations which come from your ankles, legs, pelvis, abdomen, chest, neck, shoulders, arms, jaw, face, eyes. Ask yourself if these areas feel good, bad, relaxed, tense, warm, cold, hard, or soft. In other words, do you feel ease or dis-ease?

Feel the sensations of your breathing and heart beat. Feel for sensations of relaxation, warmth, tension, numbness, pulsation, or lightness. Then notice feelings that seem to come from your mind, such as: exhilaration, joy, anxiety, confusion, fear or peace. They may also seem to be expressed as physical sensations that come from one or more specific areas of your body: brain, eyes, throat, heart, abdomen, pelvis, legs.

Simply notice whatever sensations and feelings are there. If you talk about them with a friend you will probably discover that your friend, under similar circumstances, experiences feelings in one part of his or her body while you experience your own feelings in an entirely different part of your body.

As you try the feeling pause in your life do it after a variety of situations — those in which you feel exhilarated and happy, those in which you feel uncomfortable. You will begin to recognize how thoughts and feelings are expressed in your body as physical sensations, and how actual physiological changes occur in response to your ideas and emotions.

After a short time you will find that the feeling pause is very easy to do, that you can do it almost without thinking. In fact, you may discover that it is a skill you have had all along, that it is really nothing new; you are simply using it in a more deliberate way now than you did in the past.

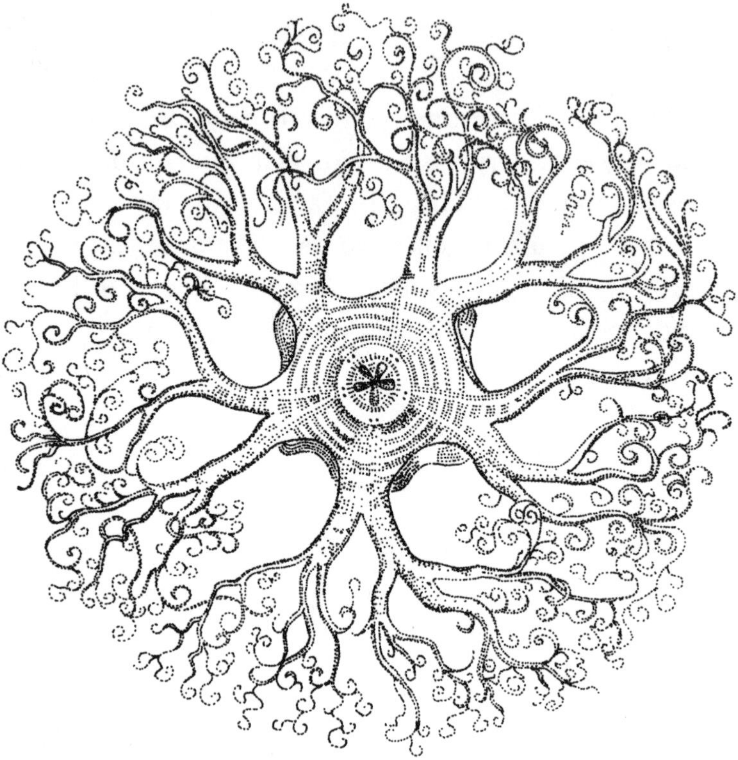

5
Your Individual Self

A multi-celled organism, a starfish, called Gorgonocephalus

When we observe the workings of the natural world in which we live, using both scientific and intuitive methods, a constant rule we discover is that it is always changing. Although it may seem like a paradox, change is necessary to create harmony. Electrons are always spinning around their nuclei, cells are always being replaced in the body, the seasons are always changing, the earth is constantly moving around the sun. These changes are expressions of the universe maintaining itself in harmony. In fact, the concept of a universe which does not change is, in scientific terms, impossible.

The universal self fully accepts change as its usual order of business. The beat of the heart, the flow of blood, the reproduction of cells, the natural cycling of body rhythms and functions go on at all times. In fact, the rate of change is itself constantly changing from moment to moment, day to day, and season to season: heart beat increases during heavy activity, slows during sleep; breathing increases with activity, slows at rest; magnetic fields of living cells change as planetary movements occur; hormonal secretions vary with menstrual cycles, sexual activity and the seasons; reproduction of cells is increased as a child grows to adulthood, then slows down at maturity; the production of natural antibodies in the bloodstream increases during illness, decreases as healing takes place; the body's need for rest varies with nervous stress; etc.

Each rate of change in the universe appears to have limits within which it operates, For example, the earth revolves around the sun approximately once every 365 days; the human heart beats at an average of between 60 and 100 beats per minute in an adult during rest or moderate activity; the human body grows to full size in approximately eighteen years. The universal self, expressing this self-regulatory principle, proceeds with the rate of change at which it can operate most smoothly and most harmoniously.

Just as there is a part of you which reflects universal rates of change, there is also a part of you which has the job of creating its own individualized rates of change. We call this part the "individual self." It is a personification of that part of you which designs and builds houses, invents calendars and clocks, arranges family schedules, creates systems for categorizing experiences, makes up the family budget, and does the myriad of other things important to business, family life and building a community.

The individual self creates or learns its own concepts of time and three-dimensional space. In our society, educating the individual self begins with pre-school children learning to sort shapes, tell time and build complex structures from simple blocks. Once these skills, and others, are learned the individual self can create new objects and ideas from whatever building materials the world presents, putting those materials into one or more of its learned concepts of space and time. It is this part of the self which provides us all with the skills to build, create and destroy. But in building, creating and destroying, the individual self must always confront the universal self and its self-regulatory principles — the changes, or rhythms which would keep the human body in harmony.

The individual self can stay in touch with the universal self by communicating through the feeling pause we described in the previous chapter. When you do this you can make decisions to use the skills of your individual self for creating schedules, situations or structures which are in harmony with universal principles. For example, let's say that a housewife has created a way of life in which she feels comfortable and in harmony. She is able to spend her time doing things which she, in particular, fully enjoys: cooking, gardening and working with children. The amount of time she spends in each of these activities feels good to her. Then the housewife begins to feel the need in her life for meeting new people and doing work at a community level.

She has had formal education in sociology and had always been interested in the growth of the area in which she lives. She found that she was faced with a decision: should she become involved with a local zoning and planning group? When she thought about it she imagined what it would be like to attend meetings and work out community decisions with other people. It felt good to her. So she became involved with the group. And along with doing her other home activities she felt fulfilled.

The good feelings which this person experienced when she first thought about community work was a message from her universal self. By trusting these feelings her individual self was able to create a way of life in harmony with her universal self. The creations of the individual self were compatible with her self-regulatory principles.

The individual self can also make the body do things that it would not do if it were following the universal self: stay awake for three days in a row, eat foods which cause physical discomfort, pull a muscle while lifting too great a weight, or otherwise stretch the body's natural limits.

For example, let's say that you are a carpenter building a house for someone, and you have agreed to build it in two months. Your individual self makes this decision without regard for your universal self. You calcualte that you can complete the house on schedule by working ten hours per day every day for the next two months. After six weeks work, you awaken one morning feeling very strongly that you would like to take your family for a trip to the mountains. Your individual self, however, reminds you that you've got a house to build. So you go to work and put in your ten hours. Distracted throughout the day, you get very little work done. The next day you are even more distracted and disinterested in working, and by the fourth day you have fallen further behind schedule. Your individual self urges you on in spite of the fact that you feel anxious, tired, and irritable. Each morning when you awaken your body feels worse than the day before. Finally you awaken one morning with a headache, a sore throat, and a fever.

In this example, your individual self imposed an order upon your life in the decision to work ten hours a day for two months. Your individual self forced your body to do the work regardless of the fact that your body felt uncomfortable with the plan. On the morning you awoke wanting to go to the mountains your universal self was telling you that your body wanted a change — in this case, probably rest and relaxation. The reasons may have been that your body needed rest to regain its energy, or that there was a problem on your mind which needed attention — or there may have been any number of reasons. In any case, your individual self refused to allow those changes. Your body responded first by getting an idea, then by being distracted, then by being anxious, tired, and irritable, and finally by getting a headache, sore throat and fever.

To relate this hypothetical experience to the Ease-Disease scale from Chapter 2:

EASE ☆ DIS—EASE
1 2 3 4 5 6 7 8 9 10 11 12

you would say that the idea to change your work schedule and take your family to the mountains lay somewhere between 3 and 4. At the point when you felt distracted, anxious and tired, you had begun moving through the scale from 4 to 7, until your sore throat and fever brought you into the higher end of the dis-ease scale.

Dis-ease is a strong demand for change. In other words, on the day that you (as the carpenter) wake up sick, and can't even get out to the car to go to work, you must rest. And by resting, of course, you change the order (the ten-hour-a-day schedule) which your individual self had created to finish the job on time.

Illness, however, *is a late signal for change.* The earliest signal was hardly more than a gentle tap on the shoulder. It was when you awoke with the idea that it would be nice to take your family to the mountains. Later the signals became stronger, with accompanying discomfort. Finally you had to accept the fact that you were sick. Does this mean that you should have dropped everything and run off to the mountains? Perhaps not. Maybe all your body needed was the rest which it could have gotten if you had enjoyed the experience of lying in bed one morning *imagining the sensations* of being in the mountains, or simply idling away time reading magazines and watching TV. There are measurable physiological changes which take place in the human body when you rest in this way: blood pressure lowers, muscular tensions relax, and brain waves move into states similar to dreaming or meditation states. Or, maybe by staying home from work one day, you would have satisfied whatever it was your universal self was trying to tell you to do. There are probably an infinite number of things a person can do, changes they can make, to put themselves back into harmony with universal principles.

We all create our own world the best we can. Your creations are very often based on things you have learned, on habits and needs perceived only by the individual self. The need to create a world that includes the requirements of the universal self is not commonly taught to us by our culture. But we believe that the more a person learns to include the needs of the universal self in his or her life, the more comfortable that person will be.

Accepting change can be very difficult for that part of us which we call the individual self. It can seem at times almost contrary to our nature. To understand this you have only to go back to our previous example of planning a trip to the mountains. On the day you are to begin the trip you first imagine or picture what it will be like. You then concentrate on your mental picture long enough to make out a shopping list of things to buy and as a way to schedule your actions for the day. You can become quite attached to those plans, feeling that it is necessary to fulfill them in order to have a successful trip. Shopping lists and time schedules are important mental tools which the individual self uses to make sure the trip takes place. By doing this the individual self creates a system which disregards the possibility that other changes will occur between the time the plan is perceived in the morning and the time you reach the top of the mountain the next day.

To the degree that a person adheres to their original plans, rather than responding to changes signaled by the universal self along the way, they disregard the importance of universal principles. But the paradox is that adhering to the plans of the individual self also helps to make the trip to the mountains a success.

The earliest signal for change usually comes in the form of an idea or a feeling. It is at this time, prior to having committed yourself to any actions, plans, involvements with other people or things in the world, and before any significant changes have taken place in your body, that responding to change is easiest. At this level, change involves only your ideas. It requires contacting your universal self, through the feeling pause, to guide you in creating a world more in harmony.

When you feel yourself resisting change, as the carpenter in our example did when he or she continued working after becoming uncomfortable and anxious, what can you do to free yourself to accept change? In our own lives we first try to recognize the source of our resistance. It comes from our individual self. The resistance to change, we feel is perfectly natural. But we remind ourselves that we do not have to act out every part of our pre-conceived plan; we can get new material for altering the plan by doing a *feeling pause,* listening to the universal self, and then *re*creating our world to incorporate this new material. We have discovered, after doing this for some time, that the universe is constantly presenting new material for improving upon the original plan made up by our individual self. There is actually less threat in relinquishing or changing our plans than in remaining attached to them!

Out of this comes a simple principle: *The earlier we are able to detect the signals for change the easier it is to act on these signals.*

A later signal for change might come in the form of sore throat and a headache. These symptoms have occurred only after you ignored earlier signals for change and committed yourself to actions, plans and involvements with other people and things in the world. The sore throat and headache are evidence that actual changes have taken place in your body. Changes in the temperature of the membranes in the back of the throat have created an environment for the growth of bacteria, producing the characteristic soreness and redness of sore throat. Changes in blood flow in the head have caused muscle spasms around nerves, creating the characteristics of headache. It will require a great deal of energy to make changes for ease and harmony now; you might have to switch work schedules, contact people who might be affected by your absence, and make arrangements for staying home. Your body must produce millions of white cells, synthesize complex anti-body molecules, re-direct blood flow, build connective tissue walls around infected areas, raise the body temperature which results in an alteration of the acid-base balance and general bio-chemistry of your body — and, all this takes a large amount of energy. It is interesting to note that in order to cure a cold it takes as much energy as it would normally take you to walk ten miles with a backpack. The processes that your body goes through to heal a cold are incredibly complicated; but if allowed to do so your universal self does them all without your having to even think about it.

The decision to change an idea in order to achieve harmony, rather than to wait for signals of tension or soreness, is true "preventive medicine." It is a decision made by the individual self to pay attention to the universal self.

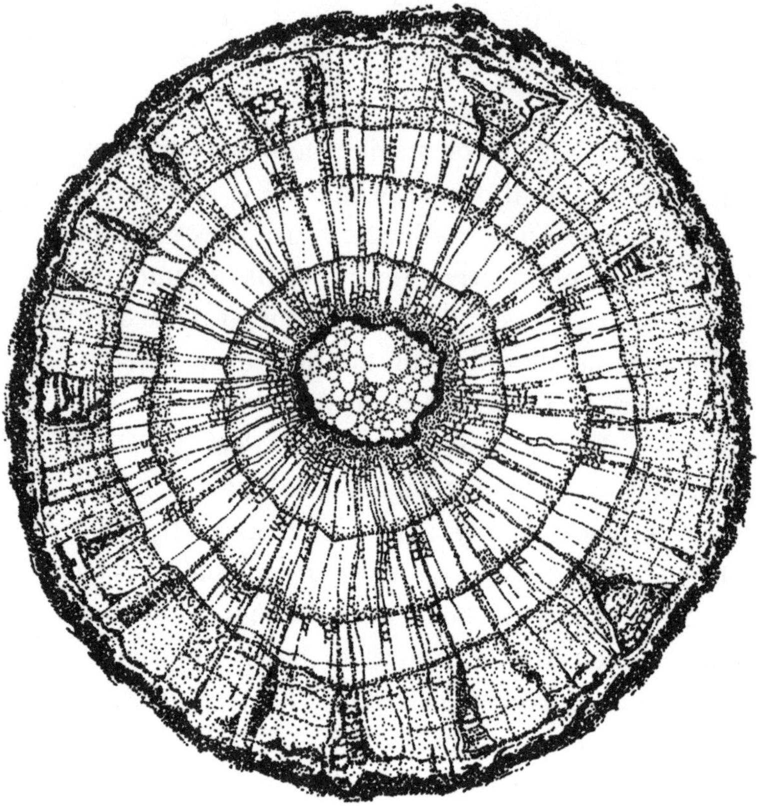

6
Making The Decision To Be Well

A cross-section through a plant stem

The decision to be well is the first step in creating ease rather than dis-ease. The decision is a conscious mental act. You begin with it in the same way that you might begin a trip to the mountains. You make plans. If you will remember back to a trip you took and thoroughly enjoyed, you will probably remember that you felt very good when you first got the idea for the trip. It is the same whether you got the idea yourself or the idea was suggested by a friend. Feeling good in response to the idea is the important point here. It is a feeling coming from that part which we have called the universal self. When you look back on it, that good idea seemed to take up no space in your life and required very little energy. Yet it resulted in changing your life from the daily routines of familiar surroundings and activities, taking you to a whole new environment in which you experienced new activities, sensations, feelings and thoughts.

For many people, going on a trip is a renewing process. They leave fatigue, tension, worries, aggravations and other feelings of disease behind them. After a vacation a person returns feeling as though he or she is a "new person" — with a new body and a new mind. His or her body, as a result of increased physical exercise, relaxation and sun, has actually changed its physiology. His or her mind, as a result of hours of relaxation, daydreaming, and refreshing ideas and sights, feels peaceful; new neurological pathways have been created.

Just as the idea for a vacation trip can result in vast physiological changes in your body, so your decision (idea) to *be well* can result in health and harmony. And just as there are many steps, which come "automatically" and with great pleasure, between your decision to go on a vacation and the actual vacation, so there are steps between the decision to be well and actually being well.

We believe that this process is similar to planting a seed. The seed itself takes up an insignificant amount of space in your hand, and looking at it you find it difficult to imagine that anything could ever come from it. You put it in the ground, water it, but can see nothing happening. As you nurture the seed at this stage, you are motivated only by your trust. You see very little occurring. But past experience suggests that the process will prove fruitful. From the planting of the seed a natural process begins to occur. The seed sprouts, grows to maturity, and finally provides you with food or flowers. Your trust is rewarded.

You can make the decision to be well. You can decide to create ease in your life. But like the example of planting a seed, making the decision is the first, though an extremely important, step in a natural growth process. For example, a person who has always had rough, red, sometimes mildly irritated skin, makes the decision to be well. He or she plants the idea to create new skin which will be smooth, clear and comfortable. In the beginning that is the only thing he or she does. Immediately after making the decision to be well the person might not feel any change. Time passes and he or she meets someone, seemingly by accident, who tells him or her that certain soaps can remove natural, protective oils (called the mantle) from the skin. Meeting the person with information about soaps may have seemed like an accident. But just as a person feeling exhilaration and joy tends to notice and participate in situations harmonious to those feelings, so a person who has made the decision to be well tends to notice and participate in situations to help them do that. These are examples of creating your world. The person finds that this new idea about soap feels good to them and he or she begins exploring what it might mean. He or she looks at different kinds of soaps and discovers some which are milder than the ones used all his or her life. The person starts using this new soap. At first he or she can see little change. But using the new soap feels good and the person decides to trust these feelings. It takes new skin cells a number of weeks to grow. Then one day the person notices that previously red and uncomfortable skin has been replaced by a clear, smooth skin. He or she is beginning to enjoy the fruits of the original mental seed.

We have found that making a conscious decision to be well and marking that decision by an action helps to plant the mental seed which grows to become a more comfortable body, a body at ease. One way to do this is to think about an area of your life that you would like to change, an area of your life in which you'd like to experience more ease. This might be anything from the feelings of hay fever to the feelings of being nervous around strangers. Locating this area of dis-ease provides you with a concrete place to start.

At the end of this chapter you'll find two special pages. One is for listing any feelings of dis-ease which you now have. The other is for listing feelings of ease which you would like to create. To help you make the decision to be well you can turn to the *Dis-ease Feelings* page and write down whatever words come to your mind to describe your feelings of discomfort. Take your time doing this. List any words that describe the general way you feel, such as "bad, uncomfortable, unhappy," etc. Then try to list more specific feelings. A person with hay fever might list "stuffy nose, eyes itch, violent sneezing, anger, frustration about suffering, facial muscles tight, and my breathing makes me anxious." Another person, who is nervous around strangers, might list, "feel small, embarrassed, afraid I don't have anything important to say, back of my legs feel tight, burning sensations in my shoulders, butterflies in my stomach."

After completing the *Dis-ease Feelings* list, turn to the next page, which is called *Ease Feelings*. Write down whatever words come to your mind to describe those feelings of ease which you want to create in your life. These will be similar to feelings you had during moments of your life that were particularly happy and pleasant. But feel free to also list feelings which you have only imagined. Again, begin with general feelings and then list more specific ones. A person might list, "happy and free," for the more general ones and "muscles all vibrant and alive, warmness and peacefulness all through me, and easy breathing," for more specific ones.

When you have completed both of these lists, turn back to the *Dis-ease Feelings* list and read it over. Tell yourself that you want to change these feelings in your life, that you want to be well. Then turn the page to your *Ease Feelings* list. Read this one over and tell yourself that these are the feelings which you will now begin to create in your life. To start creating these feelings immediately, enjoy a deep yawn or a sigh, and imagine yourself resting. Then read over your *Ease Feelings* list again. Imagine how each of the things you have listed will feel in your body. Actually let yourself feel them. By using your imagination in this way you will make actual changes in your physiology which you can experience. These experiences are the seeds for change. Once you make the decision for ease, and experience it in your imagination, your natural impulse is to make choices in your life which will maintain that ease.

DIS-EASE FEELINGS

1.

2.

3.

4.

5.

6.

7.

EASE FEELINGS

1.

2.

3.

4.

5.

6.

7.

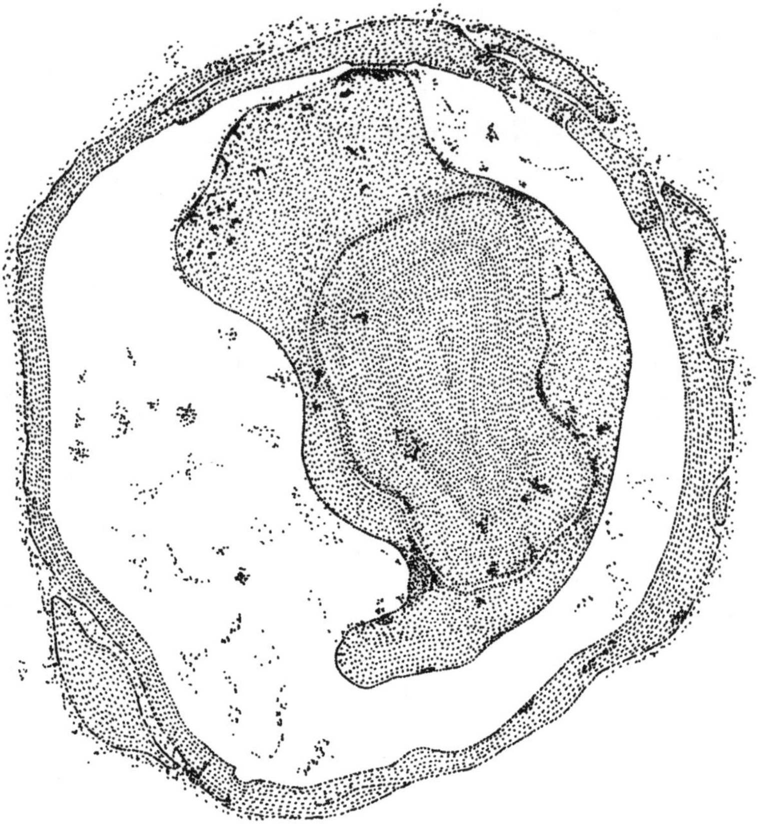

7

Ease and Dis-Ease Are Guides In Your Life

A red blood cell in a capillary, magnified about 20 thousand times

Without thinking about it, most of us have adopted attitudes which define sickness and health in very confining terms. According to these attitudes, illness seems to be something which comes from the outside and attacks us as if we were powerless victims. Once attacked there seems to be no alternative for us but to go to a physician. Many people feel the physician sees disease as a danger to the patient and an enemy that must be eradicated. Within this system it is characteristic for the physician to treat symptoms without asking the patient to find causes. The doctor might reflect on the possibility that certain bacteria are present, but does not reflect on why the person with the disease created situations in life by which he or she became host to a dis-ease-causing bacteria. And the physician usually does not shed light on what purposes (signal for change) the dis-ease might serve in the sick person's life.

This model of how healing works is not limited to the medical doctor. For example, a person with a headache goes to an herbalist who matches that person's symptoms with the symptoms of a dis-ease which that healer has studied. A certain herb is recommended and in time the symptoms disappear. Or, an acupuncturist sees a person with aching joints, matches those symptoms to ones that he or she has learned, and then applies needles to change the energy flow and erase the patient's symptoms. Or, a dietician sees a person with stomach pains, recommends certain dietary changes, and in time this patient's symptoms disappear.

In all these situations the healer takes an active role and *does something to* the sick person (who is passive). Such healers give a person who is sick a place to turn outside himself or herself, where he or she can gain power over the disease that troubles them. The sick person, in this approach to healing, does not necessarily try to understand the cause of their diseases nor is he or she expected to use their own healing abilities for understanding the cause. The passive *patient* is not asked to take an active role in the healing process.

To one degree or another it is true that a healer is a person who has special knowledge, experience, skill, equipment, power or "energy" to heal disease, at least at a symptomatic level. But every doctor knows that people heal themselves by their own healing abilities, including the abilities to produce antibodies, to mend damaged tissue, and to regenerate dying cells. And no one but the patient can create an attitude of well-being for him or herself, thus to free their self-healing abilities to work at their best.

☆ ☆ ☆

By now you will probably have gotten a fairly comfortable grasp of the new vision of dis-ease which we are proposing. We have, first of all, defined disease as a "lack of ease," rather than "something which comes from outside a person and strikes them down like a powerless victim." Being well is a dynamic movement, a process which is always changing, rather than a static state. Almost no one in the world is perfectly well at all times; we all move between relative dis-ease and ease.

A feeling of ease is, of course, a feeling that everyone enjoys. It means that a person's individual self is in relative harmony with his or her universal self. A person has a sense of well-being, confidence, positivity. His or her body is comfortable and energetic. The person feels fulfilled and at peace. The more frequently that peoples' ideas, actions and emotions are in accord with their universal selves, the greater the ease they will find in their life. The state of being perfectly well would be to experience, at all times, feelings of confidence, positivism, comfort, high energy, fulfillment, and being at peace with the world around us.

As we have previously said, the healing abilities with which all of us are born, naturally draw us toward ease. Each of those abilities contributes to the creation of a strong impulse toward well-being. It is this impulse for ease that motivates us to seek comfort when we are uncomfortable, to seek peace when we are in turmoil, to seek freedom when we feel confined, and to seek health when we feel sick. As such, this impulse to find ease is a powerful expression of the universal self.

Dis-ease (the lack of ease) is not a state which most people enjoy. It is a state from which most people want to escape. But more important than this it is a feeling which a person experiences, often with physical manifestations, when there is discord between the universal and the individual selves. All dis-ease signals the need to change, to find ways to create greater harmony between the two selves.

Ease and dis-ease, expressed in your body as feelings, give you dependable indicators for choosing changes that will make you feel better. One way to look at these expressions is this: your body is a barometer. At one end of the scale is ease, telling you about harmony. At the other end of the scale is dis-ease, telling you about disharmony. Ease and dis-ease, seen in this way, can guide you in your life in much the same way that the words ''hot'' and ''cold'' guide children in games of *hide-and-seek*; hot when you are close to your goal, cold when you are far from it and you need to seek a different course of action in order to reach you goal. You would not, using this barometer of feelings, need to know your goal before you got there; you would simply follow your body's signals. As you heeded them these feelings would help you zero in on a goal which fully satisfied you.

Dis-ease, then, need not be looked upon as an evil thing coming from outside you. On the contrary, it is *a feeling or a condition coming from inside you to tell you to alter the path you are presntly on.*

What does this mean in terms of present systems of healing which focus on removing symptoms rather than heeding the call for change? The first thing that comes to our minds is that if symptoms are always erased, if dis-eases are always destroyed, without examining those dis-eases as indicators for change, a person might never gain sight of his or her path or goal, might never be able to enjoy doing the things that could bring pleasure and personal fulfillment to his or her life. A person could continue on a path which created dis-ease for him or her over and over again, to be relieved only by temporary therapies. The manifestations of dis-ease might then become progressively worse as the body's signals became progressively more demanding. Still the person might stay on a life course which was uncomfortable, frustrating or irritating to him or her. Perhaps he or she stays in a bad job, believing he or she must make more money. Perhaps the person does nothing to examine causes of conflict to improve a marriage, because he or she is afraid of admitting to an error. All these static conditions are possible as long as people erase symptoms of dis-ease without first examining how dis-ease serves as a signal for change.

We believe that self-alienation is quite probable for people who continue to resist the changes signaled by dis-ease, since ease and dis-ease are basic mechanisms by which we are led to self-knowledge. The greater the alienation the greater is the disharmony between individual and universal selves, and the greater is the potential for manifesting dis-ease.

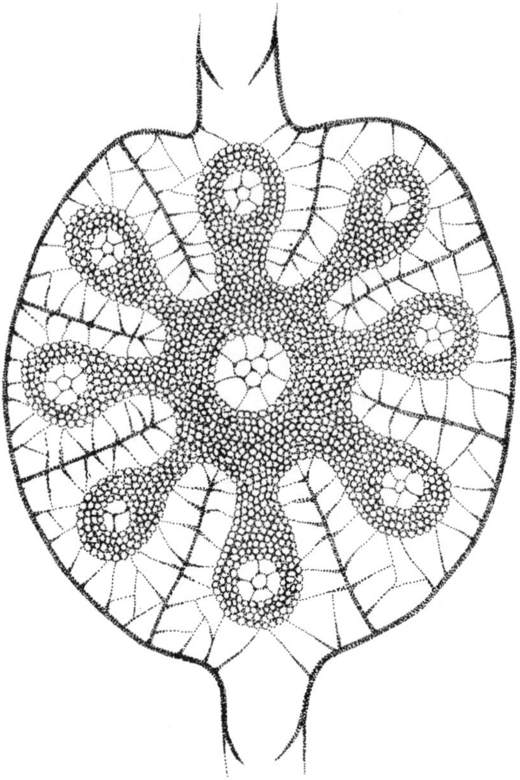

8

Preventing Dis-Ease: Using The Feeling Pause

A section through a lymph node

The feeling pause can be a key tool for preventing dis-ease. It can help you to become aware of the earliest feelings from your body and mind: feelings of ease and feelings of dis-ease. The feeling pause, used in a way which we will describe, helps you to change your idea of what it means to be *comfortable enough to feel confident about a situation in your life, or uncomfortable enough to find ways to change that situation.*

Going back to the scale of ease and dis-ease which we presented in chapter 2:

EASE					☆			DIS—EASE			
1	2	3	4	5	6	7	8	9	10	11	12

you will learn to respond to signals for change in the 4 to 6 and lower range; previously you may not have responded until the signals reached the 8 to 10 range.

By using the feeling pause to read earlier messages of ease or dis-ease, you can begin to be aware of your feelings in their germinal or "seed" stages. The metaphor here is that "from a seed a large tree can grow." You can easily choose where to plant the seed. But transplanting a full-grown tree will take a tremendous amount of energy, probably more energy than you can exert alone. The course of a seed's life, on the other hand, can easily be altered.

The parallel in your own life might go something like this: you get an idea one day that you would like to change your job situation. This is the "seed." Your feelings that you would like to make a change are confirmed by the fact that whenever you think about your present job you become uncomfortable. But you tell yourself that this is a bad time to change jobs because jobs are scarce. As you consider that problem you become even more tense than before. You begin to feel trapped. While at work one day you feel tension in your lower back, a discomfort you had in the past but which you have not experienced for a number of years.

At this point the seed idea has grown to the size of a small seedling; muscles in your lower back, around your spine, are mildly contracting, causing pressure on snall blood vessels which normally carry blood to that area. As this contraction reduces the flow of blood, fewer nutriments are brought to cells in the area. Also, these cells normally excrete waste products, just as all living things do. These wastes are beginning to accumulate in your back muscles because the flow of blood which usually carries them away is slowed by the contraction. The conditions now prevailing — the lack of nutriments and the accumulation of wastes — are communicated to you as definite feelings of dis-ease; i.e. mild pain.

As your feelings of tension and discomfort increase, you become worried and less confident in yourself. Partly because of this you decide to put off your search for a new job. The low-back pain continues to increase until one day, when bending down to pick up an object you have dropped, you experience an intense, sharp pain in your lower back. The pain is so intense that you are unable, the next day, to go to work. Instead you stay home in bed.

This situation, which began with the seed idea of wanting to change your job because it was causing you to feel discomfort, has now grown to be a small tree, manifesting itself in the dis-ease recognized as lower back pain.

Biologically what has happened is this: due to constant muscle tension over a long period of time, changes have occurred in the physiology of the lower back. The "disc" or cartilage between the vertebrae is slightly swollen and distorted, pressing on large nerves and blood vessels. These distortions have taken place because of the changes in posture created by muscle tension in that area. These conditions can be repaired by *normalizing* the area: that is, by returning it to the postures and tensions which best conform to the original shapes of healthy muscles, bones, and cartilage in the area.

When your lower back pain continues you are forced to stop the work you have been doing. You are told by your doctor that you must take two to three weeks with complete bed rest, flat on your back, to allow your body to heal itself. The doctor warns you that if the dis-ease situation persists, and you do not do anything to let the area normalize, there is no way to correct it except by surgery.

In the beginning of this series of events, the seed idea of feeling uncomfortable about your job was your first message that it was time for a change. At that point there were no physiological dis-ease manifestations in your body. A change of *ideas,* rather than physical structures, would have been all that was necessary. These options for change were probably numerous: changing the job was one, doing something to resolve conflicts in your job was another, relaxing both during and after your work day was a third. In any case, the change might have been accomplished with a relatively small amount of effort on your part. If the change had been made at this point, such a change would have constituted a preventive measure.

The conclusion is of course obvious. The closer you are to the seed stage of a dis-ease, the easier it is to *make the choice for ease* and *find something to do to create that ease*. The feeling pause gives you the ability to contact your body's messages at the very early seed stage and make changes that free your inborn healing abilities to work at their best.

☆ ☆ ☆

The feeling pause is a natural response which all of us use, without thinking about it, every day of our lives. It is a moment in which we briefly close off messages from the world around us, or *outside* us, so that we can get in touch with feelings that come from ourselves.

In many people's lives, day-to-day events demand so much attention that it's difficult for them to find the time and place to make decisions about problems of personal importance. They do not find the time to give as much attention as they would like to give to problems about their career, their style of life, or their family.

By developing your experience with the feeling pause, you can temporarily free yourself of the demands of busy day-to-day events; you can create an imaginary space in your mind where you can ask yourself far-reaching questions and get answers from your universal self to help you in making important personal decisions.

Developing the feeling pause for asking questions and getting answers is accomplished by imagining that the feeling pause is a real place, identifiable by sensations such as color, shape and touch. Actually, this is not such an unusual experience at all. Many people, when trying to solve a difficult problem, automatically let themselves remember places from their pasts where they went to be alone. One person may remember a room, another may remember a place in nature, where they felt secure and at peace. He or she might remember exactly how the place looked: colors, patterns, even smells, and tactile sensations. When they do so, they once more feel that they have all the time in the world, and the freedom to find answers to the questions which are important to them. They feel they are in a place where their questions will be answered.

Of course, not everyone has the good fortune to have a favorite place to remember and use in this way. But you can make a place like this for yourself. Creating this place in your mind will be similar to the experience of recalling the colors, shapes, and feelings of a place you once visited during a vacation trip. And, the feeling pause space will seem to become as substantial, pleasant and meaningful to you as the most pleasant event you can remember. This experience can then be used to help you develop other natural healing abilities which you have.

In order to help you accomplish these things, we searched for an image which would be outside the realm of everyday experience yet clearly a part of it. We finally discovered this image in photos and narratives brought back to Earth by our astronauts and published in newspapers and magazines across the country. What better place than outer space to imagine oneself free of the concerns of everyday life!

You will find that in the next paragraphs we have included detailed instructions for relaxing yourself. These instructions are no more than elaborations of the yawn or sigh, together with imagining yourself resting, which you read about in previous chapters. These more elaborate instructions will allow you to take yourself a little further into a relaxed and restful state. Also, for reasons we don't fully understand, the experience of imagining oneself in space seems to create feelings of tranquility, expansiveness and openness for many people. And the physiological changes which can take place during this time are similar to those measured in people who are in extremely relaxed states, or who are meditating. Before reading the descriptive passages below, you may find it helpful to recall photos you have seen in magazines and on television which show you how the earth looks from outer space.

☆ ☆ ☆

Choose a time of day and a place where you will no be disturbed. Lie down on a bed, or on the floor, or sit where you will be comfortable. Your legs and arms should not be crossed or cramped in any way.

Let your eyes be closed. Take a slow, deep breath, inhaling through your nose. Allow your chest and your abdomen to expand as you breathe. Feel the fullness of your lungs and abdomen, as they fill with air. Now hold your breath for a moment. Then exhale slowly and enjoy the feelings of the air moving out through your nostrils. Feel your chest and your abdomen relax. Take another slow, deep breath, inhaling through your nose. Enjoy the luxury of this breath as though you were inhaling the delicious scent of spring blossoms. Feel your chest and abdomen become full. Then exhale slowly, feeling your chest and abdomen relax. Do this 3 or 4 times. Now let yourself breathe normally.

Feel your feet and legs. Imagine them becoming very heavy. Imagine your buttocks, back shoulders, arms, hands, and head becoming very heavy. Imagine them being too heavy to lift. Enjoy this feeling of heaviness for a moment.

Now imagine what it would be like to move into outer space. Imagine yourself drifting weightlessly. Imagine the deep, pure blue color of space all around you. Imagine how the earth looks far in the distance.

Imagine stars and planets moving past you in the distance. Imagine yourself moving into a space of diffuse white light, as bright and ethereal as a distant star. As you approach this light, it increases in size until you feel yourself surrounded by its glow. Being in the light you feel that you are bathed in feelings of tranquility and clarity.

If disturbing thoughts or feelings enter your mind as you are in this feeling pause space, allow them to pass by you just as you imagine planets and stars passing by you on this voyage. Let these thoughts and feelings fade into the distance, leaving them behind you in the same way that you might imagine a comet disappearing over the horizon.

Stay in this mental space for as long as you wish. Enjoy it as a tranquil resting space to which you can go any time you wish. When you want to return to your everyday state of mind, simply open your eyes.

☆ ☆ ☆

The feelings of relaxing, then moving into space and being surrounded by a diffuse white light make up a subjective experience, an experience of feelings. Simply by reading the above paragraphs, you will probably find that you create a mental impression which makes the feeling pause similar to the memory you have of places where you have been. After you have experienced how it feels to imagine the feeling pause space, you can recreate the experience simply by closing your eyes. You won't have to go through the entire instructions again.

Some people have learned to return to the feeling pause space by pausing, then listening for a high-pitched, high-frequency sound, similar to *ringing* in your ears. This is the natural sound that comes from *inside* rather than *outside*, but which most of us have learned to "tune out." Once you can hear this sound, by deliberately listening for it, hearing it will help you to move quickly into your feeling pause space. Listening to the sound also has a relaxing effect on your body and mind and can help you feel tranquil when you find yourself in a busy or demanding situation.

☆ ☆ ☆

Using the feeling pause space which you have created, you can get answers about problems in your life around which you feel dis-ease. You can hear your universal self more clearly and be aware of your body's messages for change when they are very quiet, subtle and germinal. This gives you the ability to detect very early "seed" messages. Being *in your feeling pause space* also has the effect of relaxing you so that your inborn healing abilities are free to work at their best. In this respect the feeling pause space is a healing state.

As you become comfortable with using your feeling pause space, your concepts of ease and dis-ease will automatically begin to change. Where once you did not do anything about dis-ease until it became a sore throat, fever, and a stuffy head, you now acknowledge the signal for change when dis-ease is expressed in the form of an idea or a slight tension or a simple lack of ease or pleasure. You can ask questions on what to do about seed ideas before they grow past that stage.

After going into the feeling pause space, ask yourself whatever questions you want answered. For example, you might want to ask how you feel about your job. You might want to state the question aloud, you might want to write it down on a piece of paper, or you might want to just *think* the question. You may even want to imagine yourself at your job working. However you do it is fine. Ask yourself the question in the way that feels most comfortable and natural for you. However, formulating the question clearly is important since the answer will be only as clear as the question you ask.

We have said that *answers come as feelings.* Basically, there are two kinds of answers that come from your universal self: *answers from your mind,* such as joy, exhilaration, ideas and hunches, and *answers from your body,* such as tensions, aches, tingling sensations, sensations of lightness, and pulsations. We have already discussed becoming aware of some of these feelings in previous chapters. It is quite probable that both kinds of answers come simultaneously, but some people will be more sensitive to ideas and hunches, or other feelings that seem to come from their mind, while other people will be more sensitive to feelings that seem to come from their body.

Once you have formulated and asked your questions, give yourself time to receive the answer. In answer to the question, "How do I feel about my job?" for example, you might begin experiencing feelings in your body which occur on the dis-ease side of the *Ease-Dis-ease* scale. You might feel tension, aches and mild depression. The answer, then, would be that you do not feel good about your job, and these are feelings that indicate that a change is necessary. But let's say that you ask the same question and your body feels tremendously good — light, tingling and warm. This is your universal self, and feelings of ease, indicating that your job fulfills you in some ways that are very good for you.

A few pages after this one, you will find drawings of human bodies which provide seven divisions to help you locate specific body areas for receiving answers to your questions. You may find it helpful to look over these drawings and circle any areas where you know you *often* receive feelings of comfort or discomfort. To use a drawing, familiarize yourself with the seven areas and how they correspond to your own body. The most direct way to do this is to look over the drawing and, as you do so, touch or think about each area in your own body.

Once you feel familiar with the seven areas, go into your feeling pause space. Then go over each area of your own body and ask yourself how each one feels. Does the area seem to add ease and pleasure to your life or dis-ease and discomfort?

You can now tune in on any one of the seven areas of your body in much the same way that you would select a radio station or a TV channel. Remember that each area can give you messages about its state of ease of dis-ease.

Now become acquainted with the area or areas which feel good to you and which you feel bring you the greatest ease and pleasure. To do this simply think back on experiences in your life which you enjoyed and which seem to come spontaneously to your mind. For example, you might remember playing tennis as a teenager. When you think about this you feel very good. Then ask yourself what parts of your body were involved in the experience. Although you intellectually know that your whole body is involved when you play tennis, your impression can be that your greatest pleasures seem to be associated with only one body area, such as your legs.

After you have located where you experienced the greatest pleasure, go on to the areas of your body that seem to you to bring you the greatest dis-ease and dis-pleasure. For some people these body areas will be the same. For example, although you remember that you got the greatest pleasure from your legs you also remember that your muscles were sore. The areas which seem to you to be the greatest sources of ease and dis-ease, or both, are what we call *receiver areas;* that is, areas that are the strongest receptors of messages from your universal self. An example of how receiver areas can be used follows:

A particular woman discovers that she most often receives messages in her pelvic area. She recognizes that she frequently gets vaginitis, so this area is a source of dis-ease. But she also has a very satisfying sex life and sees that the same area is a strong source of ease in her life. Therefore she concludes that "area two" (see body chart) is her receiver area. How does she use this realization? She learns that "area two" is the area in which she receives the strongest and clearest messages from her universal self. In her life she pays attention to that area. She *listens* to that area, *feels* that area, and is able to receive the first subtle messages telling her of harmony, or telling her of dis-harmony and the need for change in her life. On the most practical level this skill becomes a powerful preventive medicine tool in that it allows the woman to tune in on dis-ease while it is still in tis earliest *seed stages*.

You may find it interesting to explore the various possibilities of *why* certain areas of your body can be receiver areas. The following checklist can be useful for this:

☆ Because the area is sensitive to the first earliest messages of disharmony between your universal and you individual self, allowing you to make changes at the seed or idea stage of dis-ease.

☆ Because the area is a very strong area for you, and you can control ease and dis-ease involved in it.

☆ Because your universal self is telling you to focus more of your attention on that area.

☆ Because the area is necessary to your work or to your pleasure; therefore signals of dis-ease in the area can actually stop you in your everyday routines, forcing you into situations outside your routines in order to give you time to make changes to improve your life.

As you work with this checklist you will no doubt come up with possibilities which it does not include. Trust your feelings and feel free to accept any possibilities which feel important to you.

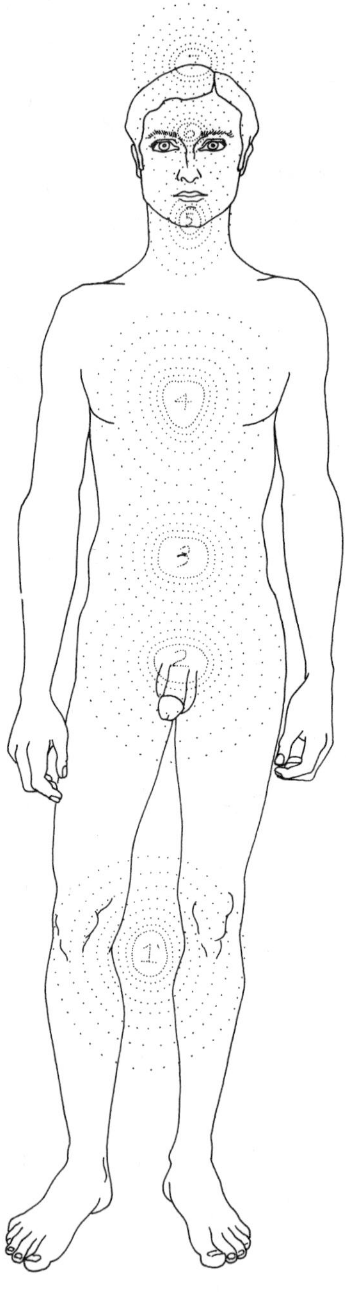
5
4
3
2
1

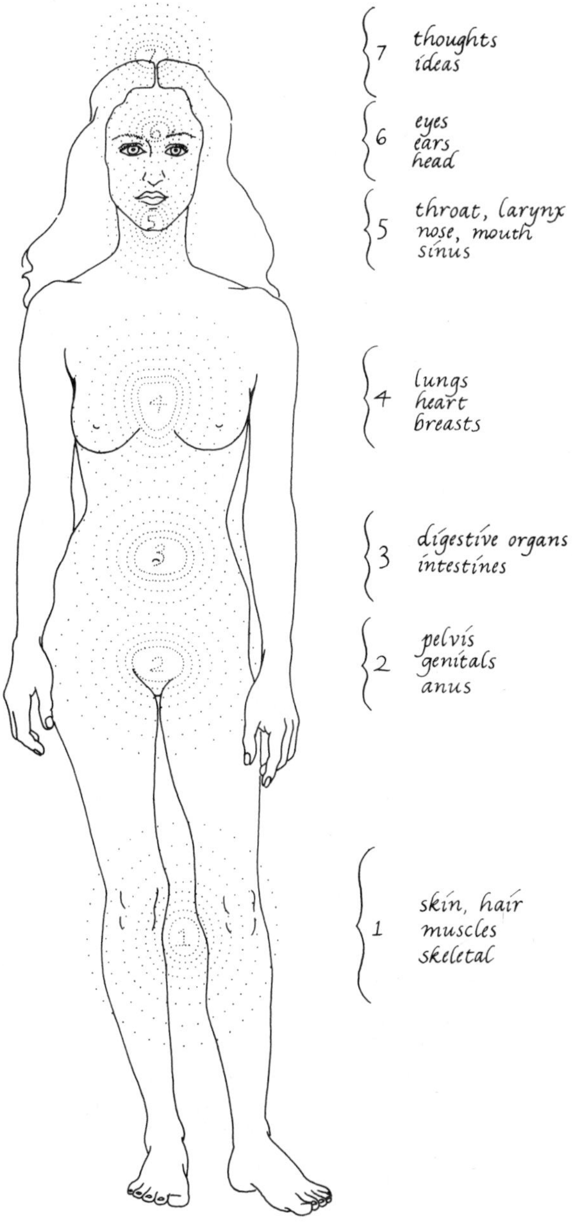
7
thoughts
ideas
6
eyes
ears
head
5
throat, larynx
nose, mouth
sinus
4
lungs
heart
breasts
3
digestive organs
intestines
2
pelvis
genitals
anus
1
skin, hair
muscles
skeletal

You may also get answers in the forms of feelings that seem to come from your mind: joy, exhilaration, ideas and *hunches*. For example, you have probably had the experience of suddenly getting an idea for how to solve a problem you have been working on for days or weeks. What usually happens is that you get an idea for a solution during a quiet moment. Or sometimes the answer comes unexpectedly, while doing something other than working on the actual problem: perhaps while washing dishes, or driving to work, or as you are just waking up in the morning. These simple moments of resolution are the kinds of experiences you can expect to get using the feeling pause. The only difference is that now you are able to create the "unexpected moments" by deliberately visiting your feeling pause space.

Let's say that a person is asking the question "Should I stay in the city or move to the country?" Once stated, this person might, in the next few days, weeks, or months, experience answers relating to their question during unexpected moments. The person might be out bicycle riding or walking or on a bus coming home from work and suddenly discover himself or herself daydreaming. The person imagines working in a garden in the country and totally enjoying the work. And he or she begins to wonder if it would be nice to move to a home where he or she could enjoy this kind of work more. This person could do a feeling pause and ask, "Is this so important to me that I should find a place to live where I can work in my garden every day?" A yes answer may come as a feeling of deep contentment or even excitement at the prospect of making this daydream a reality.

But not everyone gets answers in daydreams or imaginings such as this. An answer might also come in the form of an abstract idea. For example, let's say you are mowing your lawn one day and you suddenly get the idea that your job would improve if you rearranged your work space. You may simply "hear" the words in your head: "Work space needs to be reorganized!" At this moment you may feel as you do when you enter your feeling pause space — clear, tranquil and comfortable. Many people receive answers to their questions on a verbal level: that is, they get the idea in the form of words going through their mind. Sometimes these answers are in a kind of shorthand note to themselves, such as "Rearrange work!" or "Clear new spaces!"

You can develop the ability to receive answers whenever you wish and immediately after asking your question. First do a feeling pause. Then ask yourself your question. Wait for an answer. When the answer comes it will seem like having a conversation with yourself. There will be your question and then an answer. You will probably feel that getting the answer is no different than other everyday experiences you have of getting good ideas.

You can extend this phenomenon by feeling free to carry on these conversations with your universal self whenever you wish. Such a conversation might go like this:

Q: Am I due for a change in my work?
A. Yes. (The answer feels like getting a good idea.)

Q: Should I change jobs?
A: No.

Q: Is there a good reason to stay at my present job?
A: Yes.

Q: Should I change something in my present job to make myself feel more at ease?
A: Yes. (The idea comes that you should "spend more time on preliminary drawings.")

Q: And less on public relations?
A: Yes.

At this point you may want to double check these messages against your own body feelings. So simply ask the same question and turn your attention to the way your body feels. If the answer is right you will feel ease. If the answer is wrong, and you have to seek further, you will feel uncomfortable.

If you want to explore these conversations with yourself further, we have written a book called *Spirit Guides, Access to Inner Worlds,* published by Random House-Bookworks, 1974, which can help you do this.

When beginning to use this system of "preventive medicine" many people find that they get into their feeling pause space, and then experience either ease or dis-ease. Yet they don't know what questions to ask themselves. So we have prepared the following check list to be used to help you find areas to explore. While reading it over you will probably discover that you are more interested in some categories than others. Trust these interests. Do a feeling pause and ask yourself questions about these parts of the checklist. For example, let's say that you've gone over the checklist and felt most interested in DIET. So you do the feeling pause, then ask the question, "Would I feel better if I changed the kinds of foods I'm eating?" And you go from there.

This checklist is not meant to cover all possibilites. It is only meant to suggest areas to get you started. Since each person's questions will be different, you may have to find your own categories to work with.

When you do locate an area that feels right to work in, trust your choice. Then begin exploring the world around you for information or for other opportunities for change which relate to this area. Ways to create change in your life are as varied as people. You might even *invent* new situations. You might read something that appeals to you in a book or you might seek suggestions from other people. If the change indicated set you on a job hunt, for example, you might start asking friends about job openings which they might know about, and you might start seeking job interviews. Or you might decide to go into business for yourself.

As new possibilities arise, you can continue to use your feeling pause space to ask yourself if any potential change is the right one for you. For example, you are offered a new job. So you picture yourself going through an actual day's work in this job. If you feel good while imagining this, the job is probably right for you. If you feel uncomfortable while imagining it, seek further.

CHECKLIST OF SOME QUESTIONS

☐ JOB:

☆ Does the type of work I'm doing make me feel good?

☆ Would I feel better if I did something about relationships with fellow workers?

☆ Would changing my work space help me?

☆ Is the amount of work I do comfortable for me?

☆ Is this a good time to seek other employment?

☐ HOME:

☆ Am I happy in the place where I live?

☆ Do I need more space Less space?

☆ Would I like to spend more time with my family?

☆ Are there problems to solve with my mate?

☆ Do I want to change the amount of community involvement which I now have?

☐ PRIVACY:

☆ Do I want more time with myself? Less time?

☆ Do I feel the need to communicate with my "inner self?"

☆ Are there things I want to do in my leisure hours which I am not doing now?

☐ RELAXATION:

☆ Are there areas of tension in my body that I can learn to relax?

☆ What areas can I relax?

☐ SLEEP:

☆ Am I getting enough sleep?

☆ Can I improve my sleep area, i.e., more darkness? more quiet? warmer? cooler? change the hours I go to bed?

☐ DREAMS:

☆ Is my inner self asking to be heard in my dreams?

☆ Would remembering my dreams feel good to me?

☐ EXERCISE:

☆ Do I feel a need for more exercises?

☆ Walking ☆ Bicycling ☆ Skating ☆ Hiking ☆ Swimming

☆ Do I feel the need to relax my breathing? Breathe more deeply?

☐ REST-WORK CYCLES:

☆ Do I often get tired?

☆ Would stopping for brief rests during the day make me feel better?

☆ Am I happy with the length of my work periods?

☐ LIFE RHYTHMS:

☆ Is this present time a period of rest for me?

☆ Is this present time a period of activity for me?

☆ Do I feel that what I'm doing is in harmony with the above?

☐ DIET:

☆ Would eating alone or under calmer circumstances during my lunch hour at work feel good to me?

☆ Am I eating too much? Too little?

☆ Would I feel better if I changed the kinds of foods I'm eating?

☐ CLOTHES, SKIN FEELINGS:

☆ Do the clothes I wear feel good next to my skin?

☆ Do the soaps and other things I put on my skin make my skin feel good?

☆ Would bathing more frequently (or less frequently) make me feel better?

After you have received information using the feeling pause, begin applying any ideas for change in your everyday life. In the question and answer examples we previously discussed, the person would simply start spending more time on preliminary drawings and less on public relations. But it is worth noting here that most people don't make sudden or radical changes overnight. Attempting to do so, in fact, often causes conflicts, both for you and for the people around you. So begin changes slowly, and trust that once you make the decision to change new ideas will continuously come to you to fulfill the changes you want.

The person in the paragraphs just before the checklist might start spending *more,* but still not *all* of their time on preliminary drawings; they continue to use the feeling pause, and the conversations with their universal self, to evaluate the changes in progress and to explore new possibilities for change that will even further increase this new-found harmony with their universal self.

For example, the person spends two or three days in a row doing preliminary drawings. At the end of each day he or she feels tired but fulfilled. So the person uses the feeling pause and the imaginary-conversations to explore the meaning of his or her feelings:

Q: Did I do the right thing by working more on drawings?
A: (Person feels fulfilled, relaxed and warm immediately after asking the question, so the answer is "Yes.")

Q: Will my tiredness decrease soon?
A: Yes. (Feelings of affirmation.)

Q: So I am doing the right thing?
A: Yes. (Coming as the feeling of wanting to continue with the changes.)

After you have located areas of activity in your life that you want to change, and/or body areas that receive messages of dis-ease, you can make a decision to change them. One way to do this is to use the pages at the end of this chapter, called *Dis-ease Feelings,* and *Ease Feelings*. They are similar to the pages you found in chapter 6. But in this case you will use the method to *locate specific areas of activity in your life that you want to change*. In chapter 6 you used the same method to *make a decision to be well.*

On the *Dis-ease Feelings* page describe areas of your life which you want to change. You can locate them by using the checklist. Go into whatever details come to your mind. Also describe body feelings and the areas in which you feel them. You may find it helpful here to use the drawings which you used to locate your receiver areas.

We previously talked about the person with a backache who wanted to change their job. If this person was making the *Dis-ease Feelings* list they might write down something like the following: "Job makes me feel uncomfortable. Don't like the hours I have to work. Don't like the people I work with. Feel closed in. Always feel tense. Back hurts. I always feel tension in my back when I am emotionally uncomfortable."

Turn to the *Ease Feeling* list and imagine how you will feel *after* you make the changes. Building on the previous example, the person might write: "I am at work in my new job. I feel relaxed. I feel interested in what I am doing. I like the people I'm working with. There is a window where I can look out. I feel that my time is my own. My body feels relaxed and warm. My back feels strong and healthy. I am now able to fully relax it whenever I want."

The *Dis-ease Feelings* list describes one set of choices. The *Ease Feelings* list describes another set. If you actually make the choice to change things in your life in favor of ease, you will automatically start seeking and finding ways to improve your life. In this way you will have the power to create change and ease for yourself. You will free your self-regulatory processes and self-healing abilities to work at their best.

DIS-EASE FEELINGS
(Areas You Want To Change)

1.

2.

3.

4.

5.

6.

7.

EASE FEELINGS
(How You Want To Feel)

1.

2.

3.

4.

5.

6.

7.

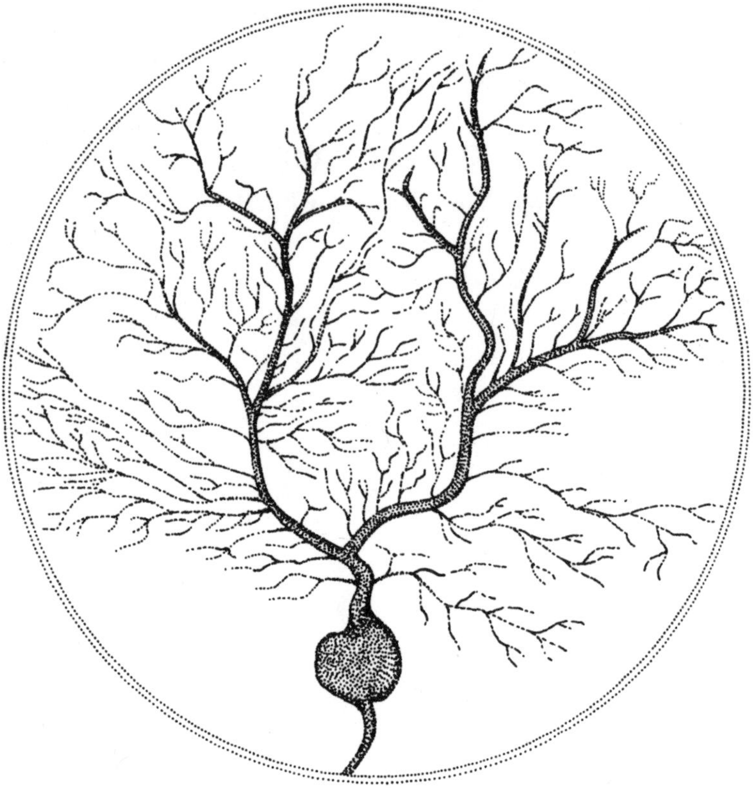

9
With Your Doctor's Help

A cell from a human brain

Let's say that you become ill. You have a fever. You are very uncomfortable. You have read about your inborn healing abilities in this book and you are interested in freeing them to work at their best. But your first feeling is that you want to visit you doctor.

Follow your feelings with the recognition that this visit to your doctor is the place to start your healing path. Look upon your doctor as a helper in your healing process. Recognize that your body's own healing abilities actually will do the healing but that they can be helped in this by a good physician. In our book, *The Well Body Book,* we tell how to use modern methods of diagnosis and treatment and how to use your doctor to your best advantage in healing specific illnesses.

We have found that everyone receives strong feelings from their universal self telling them when to seek medical help: worry, not getting well, and persistent discomfort. You may, when you are ill, want to use the feeling pause space to get in touch with these feelings, asking yourself, "Would going to the doctor be helpful to me now?" This would be a way to begin actually using the techniques you have learned in this book.

For example, you are sick with a cold. Although uncomfortable, you do not worry about the feelings of dis-ease which you are experiencing. You are very busy and feel you cannot take time off to rest. At this point you are around 5 or 6 on the *Ease-Dis-ease* scale. You understand the feelings of your cold because you have had other colds in the past.

Then you awaken one morning feeling worse than the day before. Your body aches, your throat is sore, your head aches and you have a fever. You now realize that you are in the higher end of the dis-ease scale. And you feel worried because the feelings of dis-ease which you now have are no longer as familiar to you as were your feelings with the common cold.

In the past, when you felt worried because you didn't understand what your feelings of dis-ease meant, you found that a visit to your doctor helped you. Once the doctor diagnosed you, and told you what you had, your worry was reduced. In fact, your doctor's diagnosis and personal assurance always made you feel better. In addition, the doctor prescribed medication or made other suggestions for things you could do to get over the dis-ease you had.

So, on the day that your cold becomes a sore throat and fever, you do a feeling pause and feel that you would like to have help from your doctor. You go to your doctor, who diagnoses your dis-ease as a strep-throat infection. The doctor then prescribes penicillin and explains that it is carried in your blood stream and will help your antibody system lower the number of bacteria in your body. You go home, follow the doctor's advice, take the penicillin, then also feel that you would like to use the methods you have learned in this book, to free your antibody system (one of your inborn healing abilities) to work at its best.

The feeling that you would like to help yourself may come in very subtle ways, such as remembering how you felt when you read this book many weeks or months before getting sick. Or you might find yourself quite excited as you anticipate employing one or more of the methods you have learned for relaxing and creating feelings of ease. You do a feeling pause to relax yourself and find that you feel better. Your feelings of ease indicate to you that you are freeing your inborn healing abilities to work at their best. You decide to relax yourself and go into your feeling pause space each time you take the medication which you doctor has prescribed for you.

Then you get better. You feel that you have experienced the power of your inborn healing abilities being freed to work in concert with help that you got from your doctor. You also remember that dis-ease feelings express a need for change. You feel this is just as important as healing the strep throat infection. So you go on to explore what situations in your life caused the original dis-ease or tension, and what changes you can make to improve your life and replace dis-ease with ease.

You will find, when you are experiencing feelings of dis-ease, which all of us do from time to time, that you will be able to create a healing path for yourself by combining modern medicine with the methods of creating ease which you have learned from this book. The methods you use may change at different times in your life as you naturally create or adopt new attitudes, skills and knowledge to free your healing abilities to work at their best.

Trust in your abilities that you may be well!

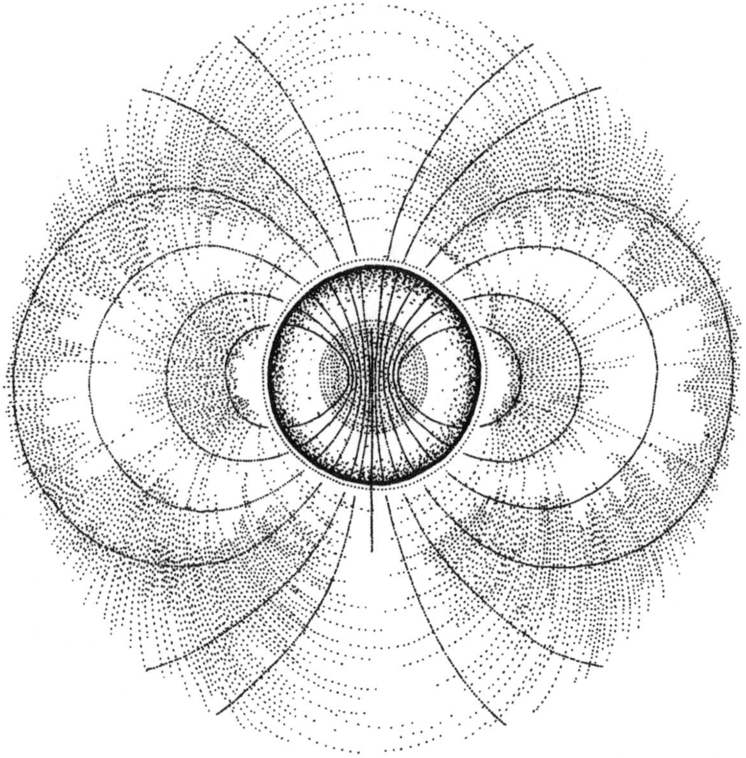

10
Using Inborn Healing Abilities: A Journal of Experiences

Electromagnetic force fields around the Earth

The following is a collection of narratives about people using their inborn healing abilities. We include these stories because each one, in its own way, demonstrates how people might use the methods described in this book, and perhaps combine them with skills which they already have or which they might learn in the future.

1

A woman who had had asthma attacks for nearly 20 year, told how she had healed herself.

She had had attacks every winter of her life and had tried many different drugs, prescribed by doctors, for relieving symptoms. But she decided that she was "no longer satisfied with relieving symptoms;" she wanted a "permanent cure."

She began by learning to listen to messages from her universal self, using instructions from *The Well Body Book* which we called "The Imaginary Doctor." (The "Imaginary Doctor" is similar to learning to listen to messages from your mind and body, as described here.) At the same time a close friend remarked to her that when she had an asthma attack her breathing seemed forced, tense and high in her chest. She tried relaxation exercises specifically directed to breathing. At first she believed that the exercises would be useless. But messages of ease from her universal self clearly encouraged her to continue. She explained how important her trust and confidence in her universal self had been. She said she would normally have been too impatient to even try the exercises. As she continued to do the exercises and explore changes she could make in her life, she discovered that there was a link between her tension, her breathing, her panic about getting wheezy, and her actual asthma attack. As she relaxed, encouraged by the feelings of ease which she experienced, she found that her asthma attacks lessened and her tension disappeared.

She says that the only times she now suffers minor relapses are when she forgets what she has learned. Then her universal self reminds her what to do, and she regains the comfort she has learned to achieve, using her own powers to heal herself. Through these skills she says that she now feels "completely cured" and "breathes beautifully."

2

One man told about healing poison oak: "This morning while I was working in my yard, I noticed that the back of my hand itched. In the afternoon I saw that a patch of skin on the back of my hand was red, slightly swollen, with small red pimple-like blisters. I knew this was poison oak. The year before I had gotten poison oak so badly that I went to the university clinic for treatment by a dermatologist.

"As soon as I noticed the blisters, I stopped work, sat down and relaxed. I told myself that I was going to heal the poison oak. I did a relaxation exercise on my hand, concentrated on feelings of ease and waited. Several seconds later, I felt tingling sensations in my fingers which I recognized as the feelings of ease from exercises I had tried when I was well.

"I concentrated on these sensations and imagined them growing stronger. I began to feel *pulsing* sensations and I noticed that the itching disappeared. I did this for several minutes. I then concentrated on the way my other hand felt. It felt healthy, comfortable, cool and relaxed. (Feelings of ease.) I then imagined this feeling could be moved to the area that itched. When I did this the hand with poison oak felt more healthy and comfortable. Whenever the itching began again I would concentrate on the sensations of the healthy hand and move these feelings to the itching area.

"For about an hour, and as I continued my other work, I would occasionally concentrate on feeling tingling and pulsating sensations. Sometimes I would also concentrate on moving the feelings of ease from one hand to the other. I would very briefly turn all my attention to the healing. When other thoughts entered my mind I would pause and allow the thoughts to pass through. Then I would go back to concentrating on the healing process.

"After about an hour, the skin which had had a rash was beginning to heal. Blisters, redness and swelling were going away. I then reflected on what message for change might have been indicated by the poison oak. I decided that I should pay more attention to externals in my environment. I planned to clear away poison oak and brush in other areas around my land. Obviously these changes would make my life simpler and more comfortable."

3

A woman told about her experiences with a pelvic inflammatory disease (bacterial infection of the tubes leading from the ovaries to the uterus). It had begun as a minor vaginal infection for which she had received medical treatment. About a month after the first onset she felt pain in her lower abdomen which a doctor diagnosed as stomach flu. She was given a prescription for an antibiotic.

Pain had continued, however, and she went back to her doctor. Again, her disease was diagnosed as intestinal flu and she was given a prescription to reduce the pain. After taking the pain drug for one day and feeling uncomfortable with the side affects, she decided she was not satisfied with the prescription and wanted to find out what was going on in her body. So she visited a clinic run by a Women's Health group. Here, a doctor diagnosed her as having pelvic inflammatory disease.

This time the woman was given a stronger antibiotic but after three days she felt no better. She talked with two or three other women who had had the same disease. She became afraid because she was told that her disease could result in sterility or surgery.

She said that she had always felt that her pelvic area was her strongest body area, and she was puzzled about why she should become sick in that area. She reflected that, for the past year, she had been trying to learn how to be more independent in her life, how to stop putting herself into the position of being "a helpless victim." She felt that getting a disease and then healing it was one sure way to experience herself both as a victim and as a person fighting her way out of that victim role. Furthermore, she felt that she had gotten the disease in her pelvic area because that was her strongest body area and was an area where she felt she possessed the knowledge and strength to heal herself.

Her knowlege both of her disease and herself was unusually complete. She read in *The Well Body Book* how relaxation of muscles around her fallopian tubes might allow a greater circulation of blood to the area of infection. It would bring in her body's own antibodies and white blood cells to reduce the infection and cleanse the area. But she decided that her body needed the additional help which the antibiotics could provide. As relaxation helped to increase blood circulation, that also meant that the *antibiotics* carried in her bloodstream would be getting to the areas where they were most needed. Based on what she already knew about yoga and relaxation, (basic methods are described in *The Well Body Book*), the woman figured out how to relax her pelvic area to encourage capillaries to open and to allow blood to flow freely in her pelvic area. She also imagined the area becoming warm, receiving her own feelings of caring and love. She combined these ideas with yoga postures, which she had previously studied, to relax.

In two or three days the woman felt much better. She felt that she had gotten over being a "victim" to the disease, that she was in control, and that she had freed her own healing abilites to heal herself. A week or so later she had a test run to determine if bacteria causing the disease were still present. Lab tests showed that she was completely healed. She returned to her job and her usual life patterns and had no further problem. Thereafter, she felt that she had learned how to prevent herself from becoming a victim of disease. She knew what changes to make in her life to become increasingly self-sufficient.

4

A man described how his son relieved a toxic sunburn reaction:

"We were away for a weekend of skiing, and

on the second morning my son, who is nine, woke up with a red, swollen face. We started to go to breakfast, but he began crying because his face hurt so much. Being fair-skinned he had had trouble in the past with toxic sunburn reactions and also poison oak. More than once he had been treated by doctors with steroids to take down the swelling.

"My son had been using relaxation exercises and meditation as tools for easing everything from birthday party stomach aches to anger and overexcitement following hassles with neighborhood kids. The whole family had learned these techniques through *The Well Body Book* but I had not realized how seriously my son had taken them. So he immediately thought about "doing a relaxation," as he called it, on his face. We sat down together and figured out that we'd concentrate on parts of his face that felt good and then he would imagine those feelings spreading to the skin that was sore.

"My son lay down on the bed and did a total body relaxation. Then he concentrated on bringing feelings of healthy skin, from his forehead which had been protected from the sun by his hat, down toward his mouth. He also imagined the good feelings of the skin on his chest and neck spreading toward his mouth. I sat beside him and told him when the redness started to go away.

"In about ten minutes or so, I saw the redness reducing around his eyes. I told him this and he seemed pleased. He didn't talk but seemed deeply relaxed as he concentrated on the process of moving his feelings.

"As I watched, the redness began to go down on his upper neck and chin. The normal color was returning. In 20 or 30 minutes there was only a small area around his mouth that was still red. When I told him this he jumped up and ran to the mirror in the bathroom."

"Okay," he said. "Let's go."

"Don't you want to finish the job?" I asked.

He shrugged. "This is enough. I want to keep some so the kids will know I've been somewhere when we get back home."

"We went to breakfast and my son's sunburn was healed enough to ski comfortably for several hours that day before we drove home."

5

A man tells about healing the flu:

"The weather had been gray and cold, and everyone I knew was either fighting off the flu or sick in bed with it. I thought I was doing pretty well because I hadn't even had a bad cold. Then there was a week when everything seemed to go wrong — at work, at home, everywhere. And I stopped paying attention to how my body felt, except that I was feeling tired and upset.

"I had a minor cold for awhile. I still didn't do anything about it but kept on working. As I look back on it I see that I was just letting everything pile up. I wasn't even trying to solve any of the problems I was having. It was draining my energy but I wasn't taking the time to do anything about it.

"So I woke up one morning feeling too sick to do anything. My throat was raspy, my nose stuffy, my head and neck ached . . . I was sure I had the flu that everyone else had, and if that was so I would be laid up for at least a week, maybe two. I took my temperature and had a fever of 101°.

"I really didn't want to be sick. I don't enjoy it at all, except for maybe once or twice a year when I want to take off for a day or so and just lay in bed and be waited on. But this case of the flu was really uncomfortable and there wasn't any way in the world that I could enjoy having it.

"I just lay in bed and rested, and let my mind wander for most of the morning. I began to think about some things I could do to solve some of the problems that had been bothering me. It was good to have the time to spend on that, and I felt a lot better, in a way, after I figured out some solutions to try.

"I remembered about what Dr. Samuels and Hal Bennett said about creating feelings of ease to free a person's inborn healing abilities, and I decided to try this on my cold. I had created my own feeling pause space in the past, so I did that now and felt better. While I was doing that, I also realized that I felt very good in my legs, and all the way up to my waist. So I decided to concentrate on these feelings rather than on my feelings of discomfort. I worked on this for about 15 minutes and I was surprised to find that it really did make me feel better. I did this again in about two hours and again after that.

"One time while I was relaxing and being in the feeling pause space I had a feeling that my insides were very strong and vital and alive — sort of the epitomy of health, the same way I feel after a good run. It was a good feeling. And I could feel it all through my body. So I concentrated on these feelings of ease and health off and on throughout the day. I also concentrated on it that night when I went to sleep. And I told myself that when I woke up I would be well.

"The following morning I took my temperature and it was completely normal. Although I felt tired I no longer felt sick in any way. I felt the way I usually do after I've been sick for a very long time and then wake up one morning feeling well. It's a funny sort of comfortable itching feeling, as though your whole insides are healing. So, even though I knew I was well, I stayed in bed and just enjoyed myself — reading, writing long overdue letters to friends, and listening to the radio. I felt really good, and the day after that I was back at work."

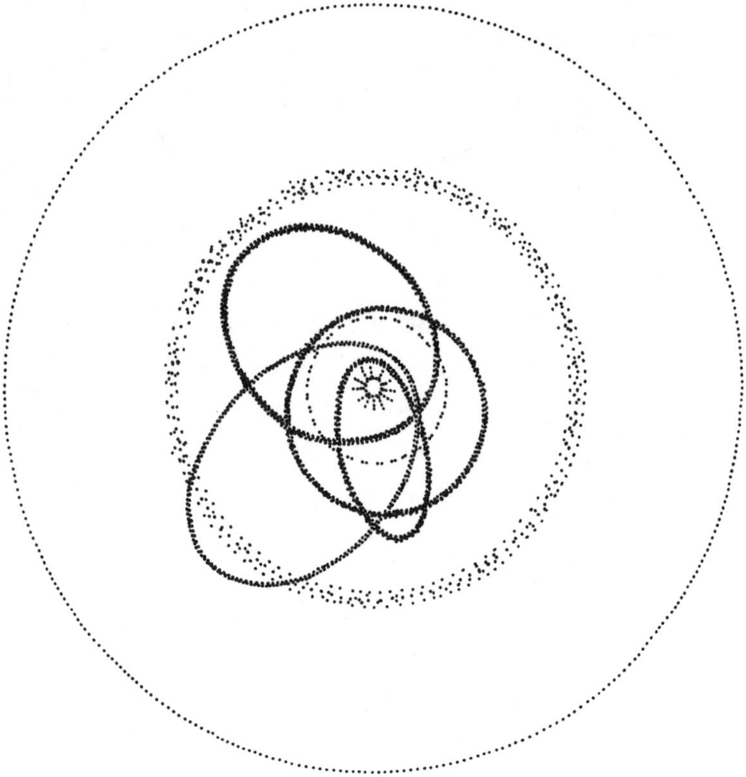

11
Going Further

Orbits of asteroids around the sun

In the past few years, research at Menninger Clinic, Rockefeller Institute, and Harvard Medical School, has shown that a person can influence his or her own heart beat, blood pressure, blood oxygenation, hormonal secreations, skin temperature and acid-base balance, through the use of inborn healing abilities. This research has used relaxation, meditation, imagination, and biofeedback techniques similar to methods which we describe in this book. This knowledge, that we can improve our physiological well-being by using our inborn healing abilities, is presently finding practical applications in the clinical treatment of such diverse diseases as migraines, hypertension and cancer. The treatment of heart disease, by altering one's behavior, is described in a book called *Type A Behavior and Your Heart,* by Drs. Friedman and Rosenman.

The following is a basic method for relaxing yourself. It elaborates on the yawn or sigh that we each do every day. Doctors use similar relaxation techniques for helping people in minor surgery, during physical exams, and in psychotherapy. If you are familiar with natural childbirth techniques, you will have some experience with how this method works.

RELAXING YOURSELF

FIND A PLACE WHERE YOU WILL NOT BE DISTURBED FOR FIFTEEN OR TWENTY MINUTES. Sit or lie down, with your legs and arms uncrossed, in a comfortable place. If you have previously created your own feeling pause space, simply go into that space now. Close your eyes and take several slow, deep breaths, letting your abdomen rise and fall easily as you breathe.

Now say mentally to yourself, "I am relaxing my feet. My feet feel heavy, tingly and numb. My feet are now very relaxed." Say to yourself, "I am relaxing my: legs, thighs, and pelvis; abdomen and chest; back, neck and shoulders; arms, hands and fingers; base of my skull; jaw and tongue (let your jaw drop); cheeks, eyes, forehead and scalp."

Say to yourself, "My body is now deeply relaxed." Enjoy the feelings of relaxation. Feel your body become heavier and more relaxed as you breathe slowly.

Now as you breathe, say to yourself, "Ten. I am feeling very relaxed.

"Nine. More relaxed.

"Eight. More relaxed still.

"Seven. More relaxed.

"Six. Still relaxing.

"Five.

"Four.

"Three.

"Two.

"One."

As you reach "one" your body and mind are relaxed and open. Your individual self is quiet. And your universal self is expanding and filling the space of your being.

Having developed your ability to relax yourself in this way, you possess a healing tool which you can immediately begin using in your life. Let's say, for example, that you have occasional headaches or indigestion, caused by tension. In the same way that tension created these dis-eases, through messages from your mind, so you can send new messages of relaxation to create ease. By relaxing yourself in this way you free your inborn healing abilities.

Thus, if you had a headache, you would first relax yourself or you might like to go into your feeling pause space. Then you would locate an area of your body where you felt ease; let's say this area is your chest. As you relax, you would imagine the feelings in your chest flowing up your body, over your shoulders, and up the back of your neck to your head. You might imagine these feelings as warm sensations that move through your body.

Similarly, a person with a cold might want to

move feelings of ease from their legs and arms to their chest, throat and sinuses. Again, they might find it helpful to imagine the feelings of ease as warm sensations moving through their arms, up through their body, to their chest, throat and sinuses.

If, as you begin to move feelings of ease from one part of your body to another, you feel your attention turning away from the feelings of ease and beginning to focus on dis-ease, pause. Then concentrate on the area of your body where you feel ease. As soon as your attention is again focused on ease, continue moving those feelings.

In the same way that you can imagine feelings of ease moving from one place to another in your body, you can also help your body relax, and free your inborn healing abilities, by imagining actual healing processes occuring. For example, if you have a sinus infection you might first imagine the passages connecting your sinuses to the back of your throat. You then imagine the passages relaxing and opening up, draining the sinus cavities. Or, after cutting your finger you imagine blood cleansing the cut and bringing nutrients to the area to build new cells. You imagine healthy new cells growing and closing up the cut.

There are various sources upon which you can draw to create clear, believable images of healing. You might want to get your images from medical models, such as theories about how antibodies work from medical books. We give pictures and scientific explanations for healing processes in THE WELL BODY BOOK. You can get similar information from most biology and physiology books.

Or you may want to invent your own images for this healing method. For example, if you have a virus infection you might imagine the viruses as tiny dots on a blackboard and then imagine yourself erasing those dots. Or you might imagine that your body possesses a unique filtering system; blood, flowing to the area around the virus-caused dis-ease, surrounds and melts the viruses and then carries the melted-down particles to the filters. As the filtering system receives these particles it reconstructs them into healthy, energy-giving nutrients which aid in the total healing process.

When you invent images for healing choose ones which describe, by your own interpretation, one of the *basic healing processes:*

☆ erasing bacteria or viruses

☆ building new cells to replace damaged ones

☆ making rough areas smooth

☆ making hot areas cool

☆ making sore areas comfortable

☆ making tense areas relax

☆ draining swollen areas (such as sinuses, boils, mild inflamation)

☆ releasing pressure from tight areas

☆ bringing blood to areas that need nutriment

☆ bringing blood to areas that need to be cleansed

☆ making areas that are too wet drier

☆ making areas that are too dry wetter

☆ bringing energy to areas that seem fatigued.

After imagining the healing processes taking place, and as you *feel* these processes beginning, you can then imagine the way the area of dis-ease looks and feels in its completely healed state. For example, you begin the process of healing a skin rash by imagining the redness fading just as the redness fades from the sky during a sunset. Then you imagine the area that had the rash as it would be in its healed state. You imagine the skin being smooth, dry, supple, vibrant and soft. With a sore throat you might imagine tiny bacteria becoming crystals which your saliva dissolves; then your stomach converts these dissolved crystals to health-giving minerals which flow into your blood stream. After you start this healing process in your imagination, you then imagine the mucous membrane in the back of your throat becoming pink, slightly moist and feeling very comfortable, just as it feels in its most well state.

Basic sensations of *healed states* are:

- ☆ smoothness
- ☆ comfort
- ☆ gentle warmth
- ☆ the suppleness of new tissue
- ☆ moistness (not too wet, not too dry)
- ☆ resiliency
- ☆ strength
- ☆ ease and harmony

The methods we describe here work in general ways throughout your body. They free your inborn healing abilities to operate at their best. When you are sick use these healing methods with the same regularity that would expect to use another healing method such as drugs or physical therapy. You are freeing inborn healing abilities to do their work. No healing can occur without them but you can do things to strengthen them, encourage them, and free them. You can use these methods to *help* you heal *any* dis-ease. We have found them to be especially helpful with healing common colds, hay fever, sinusitis, asthma, allergies, minor cuts and burns, muscular aches and pains, low back pain, headache, indigestion, and skin diseases such as poison oak or sunburn. You can also use them to relieve nervousness, anxiety or depression.

All these methods can be used in addition to any other treatment you may be getting. As we have mentioned, medical researchers are beginning to use similar methods as part of the treatment for many diseases, including high blood pressure, cancer and heart disease.

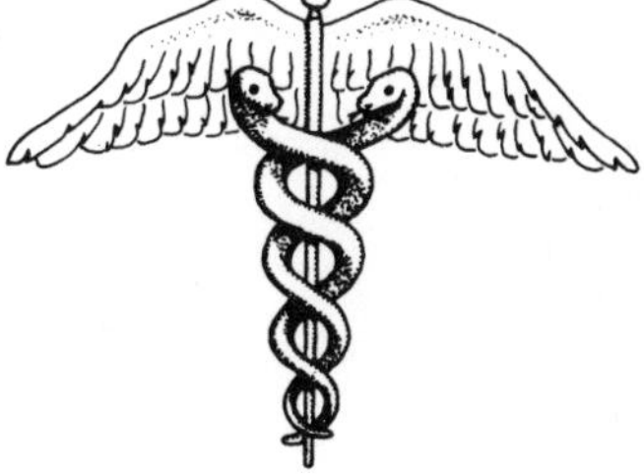

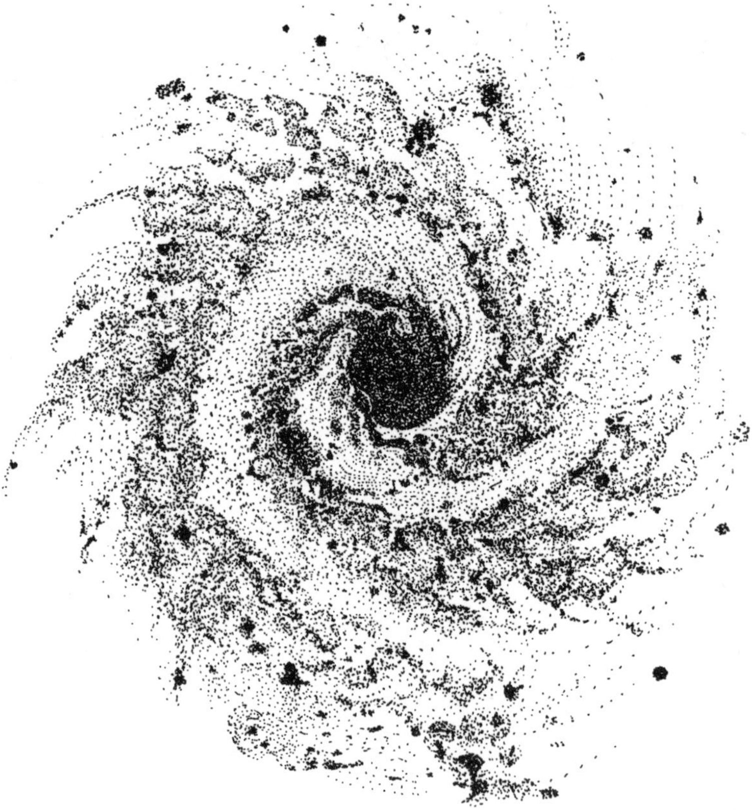

Afterword

The Milky Way galaxy

About The Authors

It is a rare and glad occasion in publishing when two writers, co-authoring a book, so clearly complement one another, as do Mike Samuels and Hal Bennett. In a book on patient education, what more could one wish for than a doctor interested in education and an educator interested in medicine? Indeed, they seem to write as though from one mind. In describing their writing relationship, they have said:

"When we get together to write, the process seems to be one of discovery. We sit down, think and talk, and as we do so new ideas emerge from a kind of mutual consciousness which our being together apparently creates."

BE WELL is the third book which the authors have written together. Dr. Mike Samuels and Hal Bennett have been writing partners since 1972. Their first book was THE WELL BODY BOOK, a home medical manual, written and illustrated in a warm and human style. It describes how to diagnose and treat common illnesses, and how to best use your physician to help with specific diseases. Following the publication of that book, they did a series of lectures for both medical professionals and non-medical groups.

Their second book is called SPIRIT GUIDES: *access to inner worlds*. In it, they tell of experiences they had while using fantasy techniques for developing their inner resources of dream, imagination and intuition, and how these are linked to healing. In the Forward, a psychiatrist tells how the book can be used to help people develop "resources for understanding ourselves."

As a solo author, Hal Bennett has written many books in the field of Education, including a

Random House-Bookworks publication called NO MORE PUBLIC SCHOOL. The latter is a manual for creating viable alternatives in Education, both public and private.

Dr. Samuels received his M.D. from New York University College of Medicine, where he also did research in Immunogenetics. After an internship in San Francisco, in General Medicine, he was a doctor in the public health services in Arizona. From Arizona, he moved back to California where he continued to practice Medicine in clinics. Based on his experiences, he believes that Medicine can grow to provide people with skills and knowledge to appreciate their own abilities and to fully participate in their own healings.

Hal Bennett is a member of the third generation of a family of practicing physicians. Perhaps inspired by stories of his grandfather, who was "the town doctor of Detroit in the 1800's," he has always been interested in the healing arts. An uncle, also a physician, no doubt played a part in spurring that interest. Although not a physician himself, Hal has studied Medicine informally for most of his life. With an extensive background in

Education, Medicine and writing, it is perhaps no coincidence that he and Dr. Samuels would combine their talents.

The authors feel that patient education is the next important step for American medicine. They believe that knowledge of the human body's healing abilities, and an awareness of current medical techniques, will give people the tools to take control of their health. Once this is accomplished better health care can be provided at a lower cost. "But most important of all," they point out, "it means feeling good in our own lives."

About The Drawings

As we were writing BE WELL, we came upon descriptions of various forms which are manifest throughout the universe. We saw that many of these were repeated in both microcosmic and macro-cosmic forms. For example, cells from the human brain (page 108) resembled the forms of trees. And microscopic force fields (page 8) resembled force fields around the

Earth (page 122). As we looked at these pictures, and considered their relationships to each other, we began to feel our own kinship with the universe.

We decided that we would have an artist friend of ours draw her interpretations of some of these universal forms. The set of drawings which Susan did for us, we feel, provides a kind of portrait of the universal forces which are a part of all of us. They suggest the shaping of the "universal self."

Each drawing, we have found, works almost like a *mandala*. That is, looking at any one of them, and recognizing its universal implícations, can have an affect similar to going into a feeling pause space. We feel in awe of the beauty and natural symmetry which each expresses.

After a few moments of relaxing and enjoying one of the drawings, we find that the day-to-day problems of the individual self seem to diminish, and the feelings of being in touch with the universal self seem to gain in strength.

We have included these drawings in the book so that you might share these experiences with us.

Observing The Ideas Of This Book and Drawing Your Own Conclusions

Many of the ideas of this book may feel correct to you. Or they may simply *interest* you. If this is so, you can directly experience how these ideas apply in your own life. The following are ways to do this:

IDEA 1:

"Your feelings guide you in making choices to prevent disease."

TO EXPERIENCE IDEA 1:

1. Learn how to feel and identify ease and dis-ease, using the feeling pause (page 42 — 45).

2. Determine what changes are indicated by ease and dis-ease in your life (pages 106 and 109).

3. Make the changes indicated.

4. Evaluate how the changes have affected you. Have they brought more ease? Do you now experience greater well-being than before?

IDEA 2:

"I can feel my body's healing abilities to work at their best."

TO EXPERIENCE IDEA 2:

1. Learn to relax and imagine feelings of ease (page 138 — 146).

2. When you feel dis-ease try this method.

3. Evaluate your experience. Compare it to other times you have been ill and have been healed.

GLOSSARY

BODY: The meeting place of the individual and the universal selves, and a barometer of feelings expressing ease or dis-ease.

CHANGE: The natural flux of the world in which we live and a tool for helping a person move toward greater ease in their life.

DIS-EASE: Feelings of disharmony; conflict or tension between individual and universal selves; can seem to be physical or mental.

EASE IMPULSE: The force which draws everything toward ease and harmony, rather than toward dis-ease and dis-harmony.

EASE: The state in which inborn healing abilities are free to work at their best; the body's feelings of harmony; feeling good; the *be well* state; the healing state.

FEELINGS: Messages from your body and mind which tell you what to do to achieve ease.

INBORN HEALING ABILITIES: "Self regulatory processes;" the human body's antibody system, and the abilities to maintain optimum heart beat, blood pressure, respiration rate, blood flow, acid-base balance, moisture, electro-magnetic properties, and body temperature.

INDIVIDUAL SELF: A personification of that part of a person which distinguishes itself as being separate and distinct from the rest of the world in which he or she lives; that part of a person which creates attachments, likes, dislikes and fears, that part which builds and destroys.

UNIVERSAL SELF: A personification of that part of a person which is always in harmony with universal law; a personification of the inborn healing abilities.